ESSENTIAL OILS EVERY DAY

ESSENTIAL OILS EVERY DAY

Rituals and Remedies for Healing, Happiness, and Beauty

Hope Gillerman

HARPER**ELIXIR**

HARPER**ELIXIR**

This book contains advice and information relating to health care. It should be used to supplement rather than replace the advice of your doctor or another trained health professional. If you know or suspect that you have a health problem, it is recommended that you seek your physician's advice before embarking on any medical program or treatment. All efforts have been made to assure the accuracy of the information contained in this book as of the date of publication. The publisher and the author disclaim liability for any medical outcomes that may occur as a result of applying the methods suggested in this book.

FIRST EDITION

Designed by Campana Design
Illustrations by Alison Oliver

Library of Congress Cataloging-in-Publication Data

Name: Gillerman, Hope.

Title: Essential oils every day : rituals and remedies for healing, happiness, and beauty / Hope Gillerman.

Description: First edition. | New York, NY : HarperElixir, 2016 | Includes bibliographical references and index.

Identifiers: LCCN 2015049479 (print) | LCCN 2015050110 (ebook) | ISBN 9780062440167 (hardcover) | ISBN 9780062440174 (e-book)

Subjects: LCSH: Essences and essential oils--Handbooks, manuals, etc.

Classification: LCC QD416.7 .G55 2016 (print) | LCC QD416.7 (ebook) | DDC 615.3/21--dc23

LC record available at http://lccn.loc.gov/2015049479

16 17 18 19 20 RRD(H) 10 9 8 7 6 5 4 3 2 1

For Joan Arnold, who nudged me along the path
with her eloquent words and her brilliant mind. Whose
healing love forever changed my life and my work.

CONTENTS

Annie is a scent professional who writes about perfumes for beauty magazines. We first met at an industry event, where she introduced herself as a die-hard fragrance fanatic. She explained she never left the house without adorning herself with a fragrance from her huge collection. She scented her body, her clothes, her hair, even her friends' homes, with the highly prized scents and candles she adored. Then she blurted out that her back was killing her!

Annie suffered from untreated chronic back pain, a result of spending her days in heels and at a desk. She also had pretty terrible allergies, which she treated with over-the-counter medications. I told her I specialized in helping people get rid of their back pain, even if they have had it for years, and I encouraged her to come for some therapeutic sessions in the Alexander Technique and aromatherapy. Annie was ready to sign up! But even though she loved scent, she explained she would be less receptive to incorporating essential oils into the sessions. When I asked why, she admitted she had always shunned essential oils, skeptical of their benefits and assuming their scents were crude compared to the masterworks of French perfumery she admired so much.

After a couple of sessions, Annie's back started feeling better. She was elated. So I encouraged her again to try some of my oils for her allergies as well as her pain, and she agreed. We started slowly. I showed her how to use an oil to help clear her sinuses and alleviate the cough she had developed in response to the allergy-inducing chemicals in many of her beloved perfumes. After a few more sessions, her breathing improved—pain is so often exacerbated by shallow breathing—and we moved on to working with a muscle-relaxing blend of oils to help further heal her back pain. With all her progress, Annie was still incredulous, saying her symptoms would normally come and go on their own, until I finally gave her an oil blend for mental clarity, stamina, and focus, which she loved.

Before she had experienced essential oils, Annie was addicted to caffeine, drinking five or more cups of coffee a day plus a few diet sodas. She told me that once she got her hands on my special "focus" blend, a mix of peppermint and lavandin essential oils to relieve tension headaches and improve mental clarity, that all changed. "I kept finding that I didn't want my midafternoon coffees," she said. "Soon I craved the peppermint sensation on the back of my neck more than my cup of joe. The essential oils were doing the job I thought the coffee was doing, only they were doing it better! I've been down to one cup a day most days and I even skip coffee sometimes. But I never skip my essential oils. They get me going in the morning, for workouts, and help me focus when I'm writing."

Once Annie experienced how well essential oils work, she was an instant devotee. Swearing me to secrecy, she confessed she was using oils in lieu of her daily dose of French *parfum*. "I almost feel like a traitor to all of my perfumes!" she whispered. I was overjoyed to see her transformation. Over the next year, I saw her shift to eating a better diet, using toxin-free beauty products, incorporating more exercise into her daily routine, and embracing a less crazy schedule—and having more fun! What I love about Annie's story is how easily she moved from knowing nothing about essential oils, except misinformation and misunderstanding, to using them so fluidly she changed the course of her health and well-being.

The Story of Essential Oils

Annie's exploration is what *Essential Oils Every Day* is all about. So many people simply haven't experienced how useful these natural, healing essences can be. Essential oils are one of the most comprehensive tools of self-care in the world and one of our oldest forms of natural medicine.

The story of essential oils begins in the ancient Near East—Mesopotamia— just over five thousand years ago. This world must have been aromatic heaven: women scented their hair with cedar-infused oil and the air was ripe with aromatic smoke from pine, spruce, juniper, and balsam incense, the rich balsam tones creating an aromatic terrain—the perfume of everyday life, rituals, ceremonies, and healing. It's no wonder then that the origin of the word "perfume" comes from the Latin *per fumus,* which means "through smoke." Ancient priests and physicians believed that incense's essential-oil-laced smoke ascended up to the gods and gave them the power to call upon healing spirits during religious practices and medical treatments.

Without distillation, the process we use now to render essential oils from plant matter, ancient practitioners were limited in how they captured essential oils. The essences were locked in wood, bark, needles, berries, petals, leaves, and resins. To release an oil, the plant was either burned, as with smoldering incense, or soaked in animal fats or seed oils. The plant-oil mixture was heated slowly, in the sun, until the essential oil had leached into the fatty substance the plant had been soaking in. These scented oils were made into balms and healing ointments for overall health, perfume, and personal care as well as for religious and healing ceremonies. I revel in this vision of a world perfectly spiced for mind, body, and spirit. Those simple concoctions were the foundation of all our perfumes, cosmetics, and cleaning and herbal healing products—all that is scented can be traced back to these early balms and incense.

The next historical evolution in essential oils and the therapeutic use of aromatic plants occurred in India, as a part of ayurvedic medicine. A five-thousand-year-old healing system still practiced today, ayurveda is based on balancing one's vital energy (prana) according to body type (dosha) and staying in harmony with the environment through meditation, exercise, diet, and lifestyle. This many-limbed system also incorporates detoxifying massage with sesame and coconut oil (panchakarma) and essential oils (including anti-inflammatory turmeric, basil, and peppermint). The ayurvedic healing aesthetic, found in both incense and aromatic personal care oils, is so beautiful that we find it echoed in our favorite perfumes today. We can thank India for giving us sandalwood and vetiver, found in many men's colognes. Heady jasmine and vanilla are hidden in the complex fragrance of Chanel No. 5. Sandalwood and jasmine ground Guerlain's Samsara, and my favorite, Hermès's Calèche, combines jasmine and citrus. I love knowing that the fragrances that capture our imaginations were originally designed to help our spirits ascend toward nirvana.

Moving forward to around 2600 BCE in Egypt, Imhotep, the designer of the first pyramid, acted as physician and priest, using essential oils in religious ceremonies, including mummification. In fact, when the first great tombs were excavated—including those of Pharaohs Tutankhamun and Queen Hatshepsut—traces of still-fragrant frankincense and myrrh were found in some of the vessels. These powerful resins are a mainstay of modern aromatherapy, used for skin care, to focus the mind, and for their strong decongestant and antifungal properties. In ancient Egypt, these substances were burned in large quantities at ceremonies, and they have become integral to spiritual practice, past and present.

Chinese herbal medicine and the use of aromatic herbs also had its origins around this time; historically, the development of Chinese medicine parallels Egyptian and ayurvedic medicine. One of the most important early Chinese medical texts is a materia medica on herbs attributed to the quasi-mythical emperor Shen Nung. In it, Shen Nung promoted the stimulating powers of ginseng; he was the first recorded person to do so. Though ginseng essential oil is too costly to extract commercially, if we did, it would make Red Bull and Starbucks unnecessary! Early Chinese healers are also responsible for introducing the beloved citrus essential oils that make us feel happy, refreshed, and calm. These are still favorite scents today. Just think of how we instinctively turn our heads to smell someone cutting open an orange, a lemon, or a lime nearby!

From archaeological remains, we also know that people were using aromatic oils in the Middle East around the same time as the Egyptians and the Chinese. In areas of southern Iran and Afghanistan, aromatic oils were found in vessels dated to 2000 BCE and in artifacts from Israel and Jordan. Both frankincense and myrrh are mentioned throughout the Bible, most famously in the story of the gift-bearing Three Wise Men, which explains why we still smell these scents in Catholic churches today. My favorite story about essential oils from the Bible features spikenard, a smoky, mysterious oil that goes back to the Egyptians. As told in the New Testament (John 12:3),

Mary Magdalene honored Christ in the days before his arrest by rubbing his feet with this costly oil, filling the house with its transporting aroma. Today, spikenard is used as a powerful sleep aid and for emotional grounding.

We also know the Greeks used essential oils, from writings by Hippocrates dated to the mid-fourth century BCE. In roughly 50 CE, the early physician Dioscorides wrote a significant herbal manual for doctors, which was the first to explain how an external application of a plant oil could penetrate so deeply it would affect the internal organs. As with other ancient cultures, the Greeks used essential oils for a number of purposes, such as narcissus for its sedating effects (which we use today very judiciously for panic attacks, since narcissus can have unpleasant side effects). We also know the Greeks used a lot of rose, which cleanses the liver, acts as a sleep aid, and can be the emotional equivalent of a teddy bear for grown-ups.

By the eleventh century, Persians, with their interest in aromatics and science, had pioneered steam distillation to isolate essential oils from plants. For the first time, essential oils were available in their purest and most potent form, boosting their therapeutic effects.

Meanwhile, as Europe was in the throes of economic and cultural decline in the Middle Ages, herbalist monks kept plant medicine knowledge alive, growing clary sage, lavender, thyme, and rosemary in their monastery gardens. In the twelfth century, German abbess Hildegard of Bingen heralded the restorative power of lavender in her herbal treatises. Gradually, distilled essential oils found their way from Persia to Europe along the spice routes, and fourteenth-century medical practitioners encouraged inhaling them, hoping to stop the spread of plague, as well as used them to fumigate plague-ridden homes. Sixteenth-century European royals applied these same antimicrobial oils to mask the substantial body odors that were the norm in a culture in which bathing was a rare occurrence.

In 1653, an English herbalist named Nicholas Culpeper articulated a system in which he matched the therapeutic capabilities of an individual plant to its outward appearance. For example, he used the yellow flowers of chamomile to treat jaundice. Even today, some of his principles—though modernized—are used in aromatherapy. For example, using Culpeper's approach, we see leaves as the part of a plant that "breathes," since they consume carbon dioxide and release oxygen. Therefore, oils that come from leaves, like eucalyptus and peppermint, will help us with breathing and clearing congestion.

In the nineteenth century, perfumers were expanding their art with synthetic fragrances. At the same time, doctors began isolating plants' chemical components for use in synthetically composed medicines, identifying these chemicals as "active ingredients." At first, pure essential oils were used alongside the new medicines, and research on their antibacterial effects began. But after the advances in germ theory in the mid-nineteenth century, and especially after the success of vaccines and antibiotics fifty to seventy-five years later, a definite shift away from natural cures occurred and modern medicine took over.

One exception to this trend was renewed interest in essential oils by a select group of scientists in the early twentieth century, including a perfumer and chemist named René-Maurice Gattefossé. Gattefossé suffered an accident in his laboratory and his hand was badly burned. He tried treating the wound with lavender oil and noticed immediate benefit. Not only did the pain of the wound subside on contact but also Gattefossé barely had a scar afterward. The oil had relieved his pain and regenerated tissue. Although he had applied the oil topically, as opposed to inhaling its aroma, Gattefossé decided to name this method of healing with aromatic plant essences "aromatherapy." His contributions to the field and practice during his lifetime included creating the first catalog of the chemical properties of essential oils. His body of work makes up a substantial part of what we know about these powerful substances today.

In addition to Gattefossé, numerous aromatherapists in modern times have developed new ways to use essential oils to heal. In the 1930s, Austrian-born biochemist Marguerite Maury figured out how to properly dilute essential oils to make synergistic blends for topical application, creating the basis for all our personal care essential oil products and a range of therapeutic applications. In 1939, Albert Couvreur published a new medical text on essential oils, updating earlier scholarship. In the Second World War, Dr. Jean Valnet used essential oils on injured soldiers due to the shortage of antibiotics in the field. And most recently, the French medical practitioner Dr. Daniel Pénoël explored the use of large doses of essential oils for eradicating infection (don't try this at home!), which has become a French medical practice, often referred to as medical aromatherapy for health professionals.

Ironically, antibiotics are being prescribed with increasing caution today, putting the pressure back on researchers to find new ways to take advantage of nature's own antimicrobials—essential oils—for food preservation and hygiene. Essential oils are finally finding their way back into our homes, offices, and makeup bags as welcome companions to both modern and holistic approaches to medicine, wellness, and beauty.

Today, essential oils are readily available in most cities and towns. In fact, they seem to be everywhere: at specialty shops, spas, yoga studios, and your neighborhood Whole Foods, where there are numerous aromatherapy lines to choose from. I love the fact that those who might not have even thought of essential oils are finding a new road to health and wellness using these potent natural healers. I feel immensely thankful to have witnessed numerous people move their lives in a positive direction with the help of essential oils—including you. With a little understanding of their properties, you will soon discover their benefits too.

Now that more people are encountering the healing potential of essential oils, they naturally have more questions about how to use them. Because I am a holistic healer, body worker, teacher, and essential oil formulator, clients, friends, and family members constantly approach me to ask about essential oils. They want to know everything, from what they can use on their children to which oils they truly need to whether oils can improve their sleep. This book will not only answer all those questions (and many more) but also demystify how to use essential oils. I'll make it easy for you to benefit from using these intoxicating, powerful scents that nature creates. If you're already using essential oils—hoorah!—I will offer up new ideas. Regardless of how much experience you have with them, I aim to teach you what you need to know in order to purchase, use, and treat yourself with as many of the oils as you would like.

Essential oils are beautiful, sensual, and evocative nature-born essences that come from powerful plants. These scents can not only relax you and help change your mood but also ultimately bring about bigger changes in your life. Wellness comes more easily when you take care of yourself, and using essential oils is a great self-care ritual. Daily check-ins will help you stay in touch with your body. Once you begin an essential oil regimen, use the times of the day when you apply oils as your self-healing moment. I hope that by the end of this book using the oils will have become instinctive for you, because exploring them is a pathway to relaxation and renewed confidence, creativity, and happiness.

This book is your introduction to the world of essential oils. In it, I offer easy options for integrating different oils into your daily life, not only for their stunning range of health benefits but also for the wonderful way these natural scents help to connect you to your breath and your senses each day. After all, why shouldn't beauty and pleasure be matched with health and self-healing?

My Story

From as early as I can remember, my senses have guided the way I relate to the world and my ability to observe the body in motion. Beyond my five senses, my highly developed somatosensory system floods my body with signals. The somatosensory system controls our perception of touch. Even though touch is considered one of the five senses, the actual *impression* of touch, of contact with the skin, stems from many different stimuli, including pressure, temperature, and vibration. The somatosensory system also controls proprioception, the body's awareness of its position and movement in space, which arises from the muscles, joints, and fasciae. All this means I feel the minutest sensations from my skin, my muscles, and my joints as I move. With my heightened body awareness, I also continually register subtle shifts in body position and movement quality in others. I even feel the earth's gravitational pull on my body. These are a dancer's tools.

Drawn into the world of music and dance at age eight, I quickly found a place to be at home: my body. I was young enough to get a good head start—I had aspirations for a long dance career—and I was old enough to be fully conscious of what I was doing, allowing me a level of discipline in my studies that only drove me to strive to achieve more. I trained my body carefully because I knew that I had found my life's work. In high school, I turned my feet in and became a modern dancer, exploring as many styles as I could: Horton, jazz, Cunningham, Martha Graham, José Limón, Afro-Cuban, and more. My training opened me up to finding my own style, and soon I was choreographing to Mozart, Monteverdi, Miles Davis, and other greats.

In college, I studied under Bessie Schönberg, a mentor to many choreographers and the namesake of the prestigious New York Dance and Performance Awards, known as the Bessies. In 1976, I moved to New York City after graduation from college and began my career as a choreographer. Downtown Manhattan was the epicenter of the art and experimental dance world. I had everything going for me: I was thriving in my career, surrounded by friends, and making my way in the world.

But, sadly, it didn't last. I began to suffer from a heartbreaking phase of untreatable sciatica that came out of nowhere. This typical sign of stress was coupled with other health issues, but the nerve pain was so severe I couldn't walk more than a few city blocks at a time, let alone dance my heart out. Condemned to rest by doctors (who claimed there was nothing wrong with me), I fought back, mustering all my willpower to return to dancing. I resolved to overcome the depression so commonly associated with chronic pain and heal completely; to be permanently healthy was my new end goal, and I worked to achieve this with a fierce determination.

My network of dancer and musician friends suggested a bevy of holistic healers for me to reach out to. I found out about a massage therapist who had trained in England and France—the homes of modern aromatherapy—and who had recently moved to the city. The key to all her healing methods was essential oils. She couldn't wait to intoxicate New York City with her therapeutic blends.

That was before stores like Origins or the Body Shop existed in the States. I'd never even heard of essential oils. I had no clue what their benefits were, and I was initially skeptical that visiting the massage therapist would help my deep muscular spasms. I'd always associated lavender with clean linens and French soap. I definitely didn't think of it as a healing botanical that could be used therapeutically. I remember thinking, *How can rubbing oil on my skin accomplish more than just making me smell good?*

I went anyway. I was desperate for relief and willing to try almost anything. The aromas wafting from her office hit me as I stepped off the elevator. After meeting my new healer, we settled in and she began to work her magic on me. As she opened one small bottle after another, I wondered, *What is she putting on me now?* My doubts and misgivings ebbed as I began to experience a kind of deep relaxation I hadn't felt in months. I suspended my curiosity, quieted my mind, and just went with the flow. I dissolved into nothingness as the nurturing oils soaked into my body. When I got up from the massage table, my mind and body felt cleansed from the inside out, as if I were starting out fresh with a new source of energy. I felt the weight of the depression lift and my hope restored. I felt *good.*

After my session, we chatted. She explained to me that essential oils are natural plant extracts, and holistic healers blend them to increase their efficacy and enhance their absorption through breathing (delivering oils to the lungs) and through topical application (applying oils to the skin). Massage was an ideal mode for deep absorption. The two-hour, mesmerizing treatment session I'd just undergone included a head-to-toe application of three essential oil blends: one for the back of my body, one for the front, and one for my face, neck, and scalp. Best of all, the healer promised that the sensation of peace and renewed clarity I felt would last a month!

As I left her apartment and reentered the harsh city terrain, I felt an invisible bubble of scent protecting me. My finely tuned somatosensory awareness started instantly processing all the new feelings I was experiencing. I noticed a sense of physical freedom I hadn't experienced in over a year. Imagine yourself, after a hectic urban workday of running in and out of meetings all over town in a constricting suit and shoes that pinch and chafe, finally coming home, changing into your softest lounge clothes, and sinking into comfy furniture. That's an inkling of what it was like to walk comfortably again. But I wasn't just comfortable and relaxed; I wasn't in *any* pain. I'd had massages before, but the efficacy and power of this one session triggered a whole new perspective on my health. After looking so long for treatments and answers, I had finally encountered proof that I had the ability to fully heal myself—and that it wouldn't be a chore. In fact, it would be sensual, luxurious. It would be heaven.

For a dancer, taking care of the body is a serious business. I learned this at a young age. No horseback riding or skiing allowed. In high school and college, I sidestepped experimenting with drugs and alcohol. Too risky. And unlike my non-dancer friends, who met after school for a Pepsi, fast food, or a Twinkie, I went to dance class and made dietary choices based on the natural foods movement of the '70s. At that time, health food stores displayed an austere array of options: leathery unsulfured apricots, roasted soybeans and nuts, and sour yogurt—all strange flavors to a palate trained by my baby-boomer mother, whose idea of greens was a few iceberg lettuce leaves next to the meat on our dinner plates. Though my dancer friends and I studied Adelle Davis books and switched to vegetarianism, we were unaware that our food choices were still way off. Starved for protein, we filled up on dairy and whole-wheat bread, and slathered everything with honey. It didn't feel good, but we thought we were doing our whole foods right.

After my life-changing aromatherapy massage treatment, I met my dancer friends for a potluck. I burst into the kitchen, announcing, "We have to stop eating so much dairy, bread, and sweets!" My friends were skeptical, since this was radical thinking for the time. But I heard a whole new voice coming out of me. It was loud and clear: my body was telling me what I truly needed. So I asked my body other questions: *Is there something really wrong with my back?* The answer was *No! So why am I in pain?* I realized I just needed to figure out where I had gone wrong in my dancing and change the way I used my muscles. Perhaps my sciatica stemmed from poor training and now I was making every step hard on my back muscles. No wonder my back was in spasm!

Needless to say, because I had gleaned so many insights and improvements just from one session, I kept up regular aromatherapy appointments as I looked for a technique to retrain my muscles. With my newfound love of essential oils, I was eager to learn more about how to use them between sessions with my healer. I was thrilled when I learned I could blend oils at home and administer them myself. I came crashing back down to earth, though, when I quickly realized that I had no clue how to get started. Here I was on my own, with only a few encyclopedic tomes on essential oils cataloging their therapeutic properties. It was intimidating. Nothing available then gave me a clear program for how to proceed on my own. I knew I should use essential oils every day, but how? I bought blends from my aromatherapist for daily home hydrotherapy treatments (baths), which worked to reduce my pain, but I wanted further access to the profound healing effects of essential oils. Unsure but undaunted, and hopelessly drawn to their beauty, I began to see as I experimented that there was an art to combining the oils that would amplify their benefits.

In yoga, you learn that injuries bring a new awareness to the practice. After discovering essential oils, I felt myself healing. With the right tools, information, and support, my recovery rate accelerated, and even chronic pain disappeared like a phantom that haunted me no more.

My next step, I learned, was to find someone to teach me the Alexander Technique, a holistic approach to healing chronic pain, developed in Britain, which is best known among performers and back-pain sufferers as the proven method for long-term pain relief. I learned how to realign my body through a series of one-on-one sessions with a certified Alexander Technique teacher and stop straining my back. Soon, this brilliant holistic method located the underlying cause of my pain: excess tension brought on by the rigid body alignment that so many dancers adopt. I continued daily treatments with my oils and learned how to repair my injury and return to dancing. I was finally cured.

With my life back in my control, I felt compelled to use my insights into the subtle world of the body to help others—not just dancers. I could show people how to rekindle their body awareness and use it as a tool for self-healing and self-knowledge. At that time, though I used essential oils for myself, all the good aromatherapy schools were in Europe. The art of blending was still out of my reach. I chose to train as a teacher of the Alexander Technique, and in 1980, I opened up a private practice in New York City, where I worked to heal my people: performing artists, musicians, and dancers—professions that are typically riddled with repetitive strain injuries—and actors with vocal challenges. These were busy times for me. I was balancing sustaining my career as an independent choreographer with keeping my private practice going. I had little time to experiment with essential oils, and I still had a lot to learn about how to work with the oils within a therapeutic context.

In 1996, I left the performing arts altogether to further hone my skills in the healing arts. Again, this was all-consuming. I watched from the sidelines as essential oils worked their way into the natural product world in the States— and as they were misunderstood as pleasant scents that if they healed at all, did so merely by a placebo effect. Then a friend asked me to concoct a signature blend for her shop in SoHo. Inspired by the challenge, I plunged back into my books and fell in love all over again, hoping to go to Europe to study.

After my private practice outgrew what I could handle on my own, I formed a holistic group practice that included acupuncturists, massage therapists, and Pilates teachers. This venture offered me a great opportunity to reach beyond the performing arts community to help people from all walks of life dealing with stress and pain. My new clients included bankers, Wall Street brokers, lawyers, journalists, social workers, and many others. Professional discourse with my colleagues revealed the chronic problems coming up with so many of our patients. They included breathing issues, an inability to manage stress, chronic tension patterns, insomnia, temporomandibular joint syndrome (TMJ), lower back pain, and foot issues (an epidemic in New York—the downside of a walking culture). Many of these were issues I couldn't address directly using the Alexander Technique. Finally, with the support of the group, I found time to work on some new essential oil blends to offer my patients to heal themselves in between sessions.

My clients loved the oils' relaxing effects but weren't quite satisfied with their efficacy (and neither was I!). The acupuncturists in my practice pushed me to take another look at essential oils through the lens of Traditional Chinese Medicine (TCM). Soon after, I was introduced to Jeffrey Yuen, a Taoist monk, an herbalist, the renowned training acupuncturist at the Swedish Institute College of Health Sciences, and the lead instructor at his own Ambrosia Foundation, which was close by in Chinatown. This I could do!

Even though I had no training as an acupuncturist, Jeffrey's explanation of the dynamics of qi resonated with me. In TCM, qi is the life-giving force generated by the tension constantly at play between the opposite energies of yin and yang. This idea synced with my understanding of the dynamics of the body in motion. In dancing, the effect of movement is controlled by shifting between heavy and light, strong and effortless, expansive and contracting. After learning about qi, I became truly inspired. I decided to train with Jeffrey and learn how the insights and practices of a three-thousand-year-old approach to healing and essential oils could better serve my clients and restore their well-being.

In 2005, I completed Jeffrey's certificate program in TCM and essential oils at the Ambrosia Foundation. (This is not to say that I have training in TCM but rather in the application of essential oils from the perspective of Chinese medicine.) Instead of treating one symptom, TCM practitioners consider the whole condition of the patient, both mentally and physically. TCM analyzes the patient's external environment as well as their lifelong physical and neurological tendencies while also considering their internal imbalances. Jeffrey explained that the use of essential oils in China drew on this same holistic approach. Healers create a synergistic blend of essential oils that work on multiple levels, targeting the *overall* health of a patient's mind, body, and spirit as well as specific symptoms. Jeffrey taught me that instead of isolating symptoms and treating them one at a time, ideally, a practitioner creates a blend that is unique to the patient, reflecting the practitioner's personal holistic approach and his or her relationship with the patient. It is a very freeing practice because there is no single solution, and the connection to the patient is paramount.

Jeffrey's training shifted my thinking so radically that I immediately reworked all my formulations. I noticed right away that I was finally achieving the results I had desired for myself so many years ago. The other important upgrade I made in 2005 was to work exclusively with organic and wild-crafted essential oils, which are untarnished by the GMOs and pesticides that can degrade the specifically balanced chemistry of each oil. It is only recently that organic essential oils have become broadly available. Even so, they are a limited resource and must be used wisely, respecting their value and natural healing powers. To overdilute them, for instance, or drop them into toxic body-care products goes against the very foundation of aromatic healing with essential oils.

With organic oils, I found there was a difference in their smell and immediate therapeutic benefits; my students noticed this too, confirming my choice to use them exclusively. My blends finally were doing what I had envisioned they could. To continue testing the formulas, I incorporated a range of remedies into my private practice and ultimately spent ten years responding to my students' feedback and honing my formulations. My patients now receive highly advanced holistic treatments, based on a nearly three-thousand-year-old essential oils healing practice combined with the Alexander Technique.

Today, staying true to the healing principles I learned from Jeffrey Yuen, I have created an integrated practice, helping not just people in pain but people looking to better manage any stress or strain in their lives. I blend together the Alexander Technique, essential oils, stress reduction, mindfulness, and everyday, practical body management techniques that help my clients adopt a more sustainable, enlivening lifestyle.

When I start with a new client, I put the ball in their court. Instead of telling them "I will fix your pain," which assumes there is something wrong with them that only I can fix, I tell them "Let's get rid of your pain. You shouldn't be living with that!" Sometimes this first shift from passive to active begins to relieve the pain right away. Then we discuss everything that is bothering them. Perhaps they are not sleeping well or they are worn out by travel or stresses at home. We discuss if they have allergies or asthma, if their breathing feels shallow, what their quality of sleep is like, how they handle stress, and what could be going on in their lives to overload their stress tolerance, even cold hands and feet. Then I have them inhale a few oils. As they inhale the oils, they start breathing more slowly and begin to relax.

After gauging their reactions and matching up the oils to their issues—we select two or three blends, a combination of essential oils that work synergistically—I go over some basic ways they can use them in their daily rituals.

Next, I analyze their movements and look at their posture so they can start to be aware of their imbalances. With their curiosity piqued, I teach them (which is why I like to call them my "students") how to track their body's movements and make subtle shifts to undo the patterns of misuse at the root of their discomfort. These are the skills they need to shed pain on their own. As they implement what they have learned, the improvements continue—and the longer they stay at it, the greater the rewards. Sure, it takes motivation, which I can supply if needed. Ultimately, by teaching my students how to see the body as a whole (the thighbone really is connected to the hipbone), their attitudes about their pain shift, and they use this new awareness to finally recover.

What I am offering with this book is a way for you to access this awareness on your own using essential oils as your personal method of holistic self-healing, especially when you need help with a chronic issue. By "holistic" I mean looking at how your body functions as a whole within the broader context of your overall health, not just fixing the part that is "broken." Both your body and mind are flexible, dynamic, alive, and seeking equilibrium. Holistic self-care is like the domino effect in reverse: once you take action, you ignite a sequence of change as the dominos right themselves. Essential oils can address breathing issues, emotional state, energy level, and muscular tension all at once, making them an ideal tool for your holistic program. Plus, they are fundamentally adaptogenic, meaning they will chemically react to what your body needs since they work differently for different people.

Whether you use the programs I outline in chapter 4 or make up your own from the techniques I offer in chapter 2, using essential oils every day can be your gateway to meaningful change, bringing you more comfort, ease, pleasure, and peace of mind.

I am passionate about essential oils because I've seen, over and over again, how using these powerful substances creates a path to optimal health and wellness. Essential oils are herbal medicine in liquid form. Not only do they alleviate symptoms; they also give us the ability to make better choices for our well-being. As they heighten our awareness, we are empowered to spend less time on autopilot and are less likely to get blindsided by an injury or a condition that seems to come out of nowhere, as I was when I was a young dancer.

Considering how long essential oils have been available to us, it is surprising how little most people know about these natural plant potions. Can essential oils help us lose weight? Can these remedies help get our kids to sleep? Do people use oils as part of prayer or meditation? Can these potions and concoctions knock out a bad flu or heal a wound faster? Can essential oils disinfect our desk at work?

The answer is yes! In this book, I'll share how using essential oils can create a bevy of benefits, from preventing and soothing illnesses to creating a more relaxed approach to life. I'll share advice on which oils to buy, how and when to use different oils (and how to combine individual scents), and most important, how using essential oils can be as easy to incorporate into your daily routine as making a cup of coffee in the morning—and, sometimes, be an even more effective way to start your day.

Let's begin!

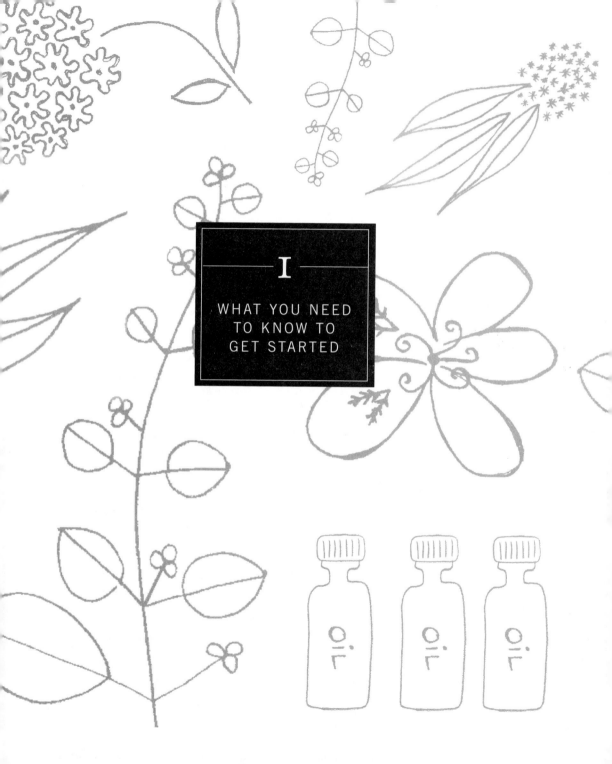

I

WHAT YOU NEED TO KNOW TO GET STARTED

In my years of training and research, every time I have taken a professional course or attended a lecture on essential oils I have been impatient to get to that moment when I can open the bottles and start experiencing them. You might be feeling this right now. It's like looking at a box of chocolates; you just want to take the lid off and snatch one. I know, the sooner you are surrounded by the intense herbal vapors, the sooner you will breathe a sigh of relief. But before we get there, I need to make sure you know some basics.

As you discovered in the introduction, essential oils are nature's oldest medicine. They are also nature's most concentrated medicine. But what does this mean? What *exactly* are essential oils? An essential oil is the naturally occurring, volatile, aromatic part that can be extracted from a very few number of plants. Plants store oils either in surface structures, as with herbaceous leaves (like lavender, petitgrain, and rosemary), or in internal structures. Plants that store oils internally store them either in sacs (such as bergamot, lemon, frankincense, and myrrh), between cells in ducts (such as fir, cedar, pine, spruce, juniper, and cypress), or within plant tissue that is unique from other cells in content and size (such as citronella, palmarosa, and patchouli).

Every species has evolved to survive. Essential oils are vital to plants and animals. Plants produce an aromatic liquid to repel predators, attract bees, fight off disease, or adapt to challenges in the plants' habitat, such as a lack of or too much water. Monkeys rub their necks with citrus fruits to get the immune-boosting effect (or antimicrobial effect) of the essential oil contained in the peel. Essential oils, once extracted, can protect us as well, especially if we don't harm the integrity of the oil during the extraction method.

Unlike dried herbal teas, or extracts (like vanilla extract or almond extract) and tinctures, both of which are extracted with alcohol, essential oils are obtained through distillation. Distillation is the preferred way that growers "harvest" essential oils from plants because it's the gentlest. It reminds me of the simplest way we can cook vegetables: by steaming, which preserves their nutritional content.

Imagine a valley in the South of France, let's say in Provence, filled with purple fields of lavender. It's a beautiful time of day, when the fields are most fragrant. That's when growers cut the flowering tops off each plant. After collecting this raw plant material, they place the harvest into large vats within their distillery. (Sometimes farmers bring huge trucks right out into the field to distill the harvest there.) Just like we steam vegetables at home, water is placed in the bottom part of the vat below the lavender and is heated to boiling. The steam that results surges up to the top of the vat and passes over the lavender. As the steam hits the lavender flowers, the essential oil is released from the thin walls of the tiny pouches within the petals. The steam continues upward to the top of the pot, where the lid traps the essential-oil-laced steam and sends it through heavily coiled tubes for cooling and then collection in another vat. Since oil doesn't dissolve in water, the essential oil naturally separates from the cooled liquid and is easily siphoned off into a glass or stainless steel receptacle from which it's poured into the smaller bottles we buy at the store. The aromatic water that remains is called the hydrosol. With only trace amounts of the essential oil, hydrosols are used for skin care, children, and for a quick spritz. *Et voilà!*

Once separated from the plant, aromatic liquids can be as thin as water or as thick as paste. Each essential oil has a fragrance that is characteristic of the plant from which it originates, whether it's sourced from the leaf (basil), the needle (pine), the flower (lavender), the bark (cedarwood), the fruit (lemon), the root (ginger), the seed (coriander), the grass (palmarosa), or the resin (frankincense).

With few exceptions, essential-oil-giving plants are not something you can easily grow in a flower bed at home. Though some plants can be harvested from a natural habitat, most are cultivated by artisanal farmers. Like winemakers, these expert growers have the experience and scientific knowledge necessary to nurture their crop from seedling to harvest to distillation to market. Each grower has a responsibility and a need to make sure their oils meet a standardized test in order to be considered authentic.

Just how concentrated are essential oils? Well, the amount of plant materials growers must distill to produce even small amounts of an essential oil is likely to shock you—because it takes a *huge* amount. That's why I call them nature's most concentrated medicine! Imagine this: to produce 1 cup—8 ounces—of lavender essential oil, a grower needs to distill *75 pounds* of freshly harvested lavender flowers. That's the equivalent of *500 clamshells of washed salad greens*!

The most concentrated essential oil of all, Bulgarian rose otto, requires *5 dozen roses* for just *1 drop* of its semiprecious oil. The following are a few examples of just how much plant matter it takes to make approximately 8 ounces of a few popular essential oils:

- Eucalyptus: 25 pounds of leaves
- Rosemary: 250 pounds of leaves
- Jasmine: 500 pounds of flowers
- Rose: 1,000 pounds of flowers

Seeing how concentrated essential oils are shows you just how potent these can be as herbal medicine. As you'll learn throughout this chapter, these powerful, naturally occurring remedies excel in their ability to help heal and create wellness on a daily basis.

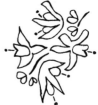

NOT ALL FRAGRANCES ARE ESSENTIAL OILS

Sometimes it pains me to hear how confusing the world of scent is to so many people, and how many people mistake, through no fault of their own, an imitation for the real thing. We all love things that smell good—that much we know. Everything—*yes, everything*—has an odor. Some odors are immediately recognizable, while some are so subtle we can't smell them. Some odors don't ever reach our noses, while others jump out at us immediately. And smell can be subjective; every person's sense of smell is calibrated a little differently.

Things that smell good can elevate our mood, arouse us, or bring us comfort. Essential oils aren't the only powerful scents in the world. Fresh-cut grass and the salty spray of the ocean are delivered to us through moisture in the air we breathe. The smell of rain comes from water molecules that hit the ground and bounce back up into the air, carrying the scent of wet earth or pavement.

The scent of an essential oil is impossible to duplicate because the oil is so complex structurally that it simply can't be broken down completely. Natural fragrance oil is more of a gray area, like any product labeled "natural." Some fragrance oils used in natural products are made from isolating the one chemical component of an essential oil that gives off its telltale scent, sometimes called an "isolate" or "natural."

But when you see chemical names like "limonene" or "geraniol" on a product label, you can be sure you're not buying the whole healing essence of the plant, and these chemical isolates may be extracted or even diluted with toxic chemicals (such as phthalates). (Check out the list on page 40 to see what *should* be on the label of a pure essential oil.) Most beauty products, home cleaning products, and perfumes are made with ingredients that have been highly processed or synthetically derived. The purpose of using a synthetic substance or a "natural" isolate in lieu of the original is to create smells and tastes that are completely consistent from batch to batch and won't change over time as the product sits on a shelf. For example, the signature smells of a product like Johnson & Johnson's baby powder or the distinct taste of a Coca-Cola (which derives its unique flavor exclusively from a heavily processed mixture of lemon, nutmeg, neroli, cinnamon, and coriander essential oils) always stay the same. In contrast, pure, authentic essential oils can change from crop to crop, making these true naturals unstable for mass production.

I'll discuss more about the differences between synthetic and natural fragrances in chapter 6. But for now, just know that not all plants that produce scent are harvested for use as an essential oil, and not all fragrances have the same efficacy or purity as the essential oils described in this book.

A Natural Prescription

Recently I attended a trade show where a young man spied my sleep remedy. He begged me for a bottle. Before I gave it to him, we discussed how he should use it. The next day, he came back disappointed, claiming, "Nothing happened." Knowing this was not the whole picture, I asked him to tell me what had happened the night before. I expected to hear the same desperate tale I always do—a story of waiting hours to fall asleep or waking too often and trying to solve life's problems with an exhausted mind. But his story was much simpler than that. He had followed my instructions exactly. He went to bed, turned off all the lights, and inhaled my sleep remedy blend from a tissue about ten to fifteen times, breathing deeply. He put the tissue aside and felt nothing at all. He didn't feel the high or the grogginess that his prescription sleep meds always produced. So he had assumed it wasn't working.

"But then what happened?" I asked.

"The next thing I knew, it was morning," he said. I simply looked back at him and shrugged. He quickly realized the essential oils had put him to sleep and worked wonderfully!

This story is a great example of why we don't always need invasive solutions to solve a chronic health problem or immediate concern. By learning how to use nature's remedies, improvements can happen without us even noticing.

So many of us rely on prescription drugs to cure allergies and other ailments. We take expensive vitamins and supplements to stay healthy every day. We take medications to help us sleep. We rely on coffee and caffeinated beverages to stay awake. I've often thought about how we jump through hoops trying to reduce our daily stress and pain, but what if we all realized there are natural products that are more powerful than herbal teas, are more authentic than vitamins, and have fewer side effects than pharmaceuticals?

Here are a few examples of what essential oils can do:

• *Relieve Aches and Pains*
We know how important it is to keep up with a weekly exercise program, yet we do nothing to prevent or heal injuries except mask pain with Advil or Tylenol. Look no further for a natural, non-steroidal, anti-inflammatory pain reliever. Essential oils do this well while also supporting muscle health, body awareness, and flexibility.

• *Alleviate Cold, Flu, and Allergy Symptoms*

Many common essential oils are powerful decongestants and expectorants for treating colds and flu and shown to be effective antifungals for allergy sufferers. In addition, many oils are antibacterial and antiviral, which helps speed recovery. Eucalyptus eases sinus congestion, and bay laurel is the perfect solution for a sore throat. Got a bad cough? Try pine to loosen it up and get it out. Antihistamines like blue (German or cape) chamomile paired with decongestant oils can work on allergy symptoms for uncommon relief.

• *Release Tension and Stress*

We treat anxiety, depression, and the symptoms of a stressful life with pharmaceuticals. Essential oils tap into the same network within our brains—the limbic system—as most antidepressants do, to help us balance emotions without any side effects.

• *Heal Wounds, Bites, and Burns*

Essential oils made history when chemist Gattefossé healed widespread burns by dipping his wound in lavender. The next time you find yourself with a deep cut—or its resulting scar—try including an antiseptic fix, like a couple of drops of lavender or helichrysum on a Band-Aid, to help heal physical wounds faster. The same goes for insect bites and other inflamed bumps.

If you begin using essential oils every day—as I describe in this book— you won't get sick as frequently, or for as long, as you do now. When I worked in a group practice, there were lots of sick people coming and going. Occasionally, I picked up a bug with symptoms that matched our patients', but I would have it for a day, while the patients would suffer for weeks with the same ailment. For anyone who feels like they get sick too often, is prone to sinus infections, or has other minor respiratory problems, essential oils are a must.

Of course, pharmaceutical and over-the-counter remedies have their place, and I don't mean to imply that these products are not helpful or important. But here's the main difference: medications, pharmaceuticals, and pain-relief drugs respond to symptoms. Essential oils are preventative: they fortify the body so we can tackle many symptoms sooner, hopefully before we need a prescription. And using them every day is luxurious; these are calming rituals for on-the-spot healing. We don't hear ourselves saying "Have you tried my new antidepressant? It smells sooooo good, and I feel better instantly!" Essential oils are an enjoyable prescription for health and wellness.

An Ounce of Prevention . . .

Essential oils have a rich history of being utilized as cures and remedies for a variety of illnesses and diseases, from the plague to the common cold. But I am recommending you use these potent substances on a daily basis to *prevent* illness. Here are some of the most important ways essential oils can help boost physical and mental wellness:

• *Provide Antiaging Antioxidants*
We look to foods, drinks, vitamins, and even pharmaceutical-grade skin care products for our daily dose of wrinkle-preventing, cancer-fighting nutrients. But essential oils pack a bigger antioxidant punch than anything we can consume, and they will make your skin glow naturally.

• *Support the Immune System*
It's a challenge to stay healthy without a boost to the body's defense system. The repeated use of antibiotics can disturb digestion and lower immunity. Children share germs in their classrooms and playgrounds, pets and pests alike carry disease, and living an international lifestyle presents tons of

opportunities to encounter a host of microscopic unfriendlies. We all know how hard it is to fight off a bug, but essential oils like tea tree and eucalyptus have got you covered! Antimicrobial essential oils (without chemicals!) have been used throughout history to fight illness and speed recovery. For example, myrrh was used as a salve for wounds as early as 1550 BCE but was also studied for its antibiotic properties in 2013. And did you know that the formula for Listerine still relies on thyme essential oil for its germ-fighting punch?

 • *Detoxify*
We want to "cleanse" when we overindulge or feel burned out. But do we ever really enjoy a protein powder or an all-juice fast? Essential oils can help the body eliminate toxins with inhalation and without depriving it of sustenance.

 • *Repel Common Household Insects and Pests*
Fleas and spiders hate peppermint, catnip drives away mosquitoes, and ticks of all sorts can't abide lemon eucalyptus. There's no need to use unpleasant toxic formulas when these plants have been fending off insects in nature for millions of years. With essential oils, you can make your own repellent spray.

Creating Healthy Self-Care Habits

We all know the benefits of a good night's sleep, a solid exercise routine, and a daily meditative practice. But rarely do we accomplish all three. It's hard to find the time and discipline to keep up with everything we ought to be doing.

Some recent writings, like Charles Duhigg's *The Power of Habit*, suggest that changing and creating better habits works best when you set an intention, repeat a ritual, and give yourself a reward. Incorporating essential oils into your daily life offers all three. By creating a self-care routine with oils every day, you'll enjoy a positive sensory experience and, over time, rewire your brain to expect and indulge in the practice of that new habit, which can translate to creating other great rituals, routines, and rewards throughout your life.

Here are some examples of self-care routines that start with essential oils:

- Deeply inhaling essential oils will improve breathing to calm your nerves and absorb more oxygen; better breathing equals more energy, focus, and overall health.
- Applying essential oils topically will increase body awareness for injury prevention and better posture.
- Anointing or diffusing essential oils will aid mindfulness and meditation practices for everything from mental focus to sleep to weight loss!

Taking Your Herbal Medicine

Recently, I attended an excellent exhibition about the history of herbal medicine at the Brooklyn Botanic Garden, where Dr. Andrew Weil, a bestselling author and one of the most popular holistic physicians in the world, gave an inspiring talk about the healing power of plants. Dr. Weil spoke about how his studies as an undergraduate majoring in botany informed his practice as a doctor. He noted that plants, unlike most medicines, are adaptogenic—meaning they have the capacity to heal and bring about changes based on what our bodies need at that moment. With all the discoveries made throughout human history about essential oils, I think this quality may be one of the most important.

You will learn more throughout this book about how essential oils are capable of adapting to our immediate issues and how that makes it easier to find success with the oils you choose. Discoveries into how essential oils work are changing the landscape for aromatherapy professionals and physicians looking into broader applications of aromatic healing. But like all alternative approaches, research on essential oils is still limited. One thing is certain: in order to reap all the healing benefits of essential oils, it's best to use the whole essential oil and to process that oil as little as possible.

The four primary ways essential oils can be administered in a holistic manner are via inhaling, diffusing, applying, and heating.

Inhaling

Inhaling an essential oil is the fastest and most effective way to experience the many therapeutic rewards an oil has to offer—and not just because of the smell (when you inhale an essential oil you absorb up to 70 percent of the vapors into your body). Every time you open a bottle of essential oil, it's like letting a genie out. Though you can't see an actual cloud of vapors, the essential oil's micro-particles evaporate into the air immediately and form a protective yet invisible antimicrobial cloud. Anyone who has smelled eucalyptus or peppermint—some of the stronger scented oils—knows how quickly the vapor from these oils can travel across a room and how intense the aroma can be.

The longer an essential oil is exposed to the air, the stronger its aromatic vapor and thus its effect on you. With every inhalation, you move the microparticles farther into your body. First, the particles travel through your nasal passages and breathing pathways, speeding through the olfactory nerves located there. The olfactory nerves terminate in the olfactory bulb and then send messages to the collection of brain structures known as the limbic system, which supports functions such as motivation, emotion, learning, and memory. In this way, inhaling essential oils can quickly affect your moods, sleep, mental acuity, and even level of pain.

Inhaling essential oils also taps into our sense of smell. Science has just begun to uncover how sophisticated that is. Our brains can identify up to ten thousand scents. This is how we know if our clothes are clean, if fruit is ripe, if the milk has gone sour. Our cataloging of scent helps us to know if there's a gas leak in our building or if the dog needs a bath. Our noses can be so specific that we can smell a thunderstorm developing. It's no wonder we say we can "smell fear" and some people can even smell snow. Essential oils also elicit memories. When you smell peppermint, for example, you may remember a candy your grandmother gave you around the holidays. You may even say to yourself "That smells like my grandmother!" It's possible to create positive experiences simply by using scents that trigger good memories.

I have spent many a night mixing up a brand-new essential oil blend to mimic the scent of a vacation to some beautiful island or country. Sometimes I even prepare a scent while I'm packing, so I can use the essential oil while traveling and then again after I get back home to remind myself of that particular trip.

In addition to the brain activity produced by inhaling essential oils, there are significant effects within other parts of the body. The microparticles you breathe in flow down your nasal passages to the absorbent tissues in your lungs (the air sacs)—right where you need these strong antimicrobial substances if you're fighting off a cold, the flu, or a respiratory infection. As we'll explore in chapter 4, oils like eucalyptus and pine are strong decongestants, and inhaling them can help resolve a cough. Inhaling specific oils regularly can even lessen asthma and allergy symptoms.

After the microparticles make their way through your lungs, they join your bloodstream and circulate through your whole body. Eventually, they are flushed out through the kidneys as well as through the lungs, the pores, and the sweat glands. Before they do, they circulate through the lymphatic system and the organs and generally improve every inch of your internal body.

One final but important benefit to inhaling essential oils on a regular basis is stabilizing the endocrine system, which produces the body's hormones that regulate everything from mood to metabolism to sleep. Recent studies have found that inhaling lavender oil for fifteen minutes from a cotton ball lowered the amount of cortisol in the bloodstream. This is significant because cortisol is the adrenal hormone our bodies produce when we respond to stress. Extended, high levels of stress—and therefore consistently high levels of cortisol—can become harmful to our health. These high levels are correlated with poor concentration, weight gain, depression, anxiety, insomnia, decreased immunity, and a reduced capacity to heal. When someone gets sick and blames it on stress, a high cortisol level is likely to be one of the culprits.

Adults aren't the only beneficiaries of inhaling essential oils. Kids and pets too only need to inhale a tiny bit of essential oil to experience its positive effects. I love seeing kids test out my blends. Whenever I'm doing an in-store event, I encourage the children to breathe in some of the scents with me while their parents shop. Give a kid a bottle of citrus oils to smell and watch them bend their heads toward the oil as if they are trying to jump right into the bottle!

Diffusing

Active inhalation is a quick process, in which a very concentrated intake of oils travels quickly to your brain, your sinuses, and your lungs. But another way to deliver essential oils to your lungs is passive inhalation, with a diffuser, which disperses oil throughout an enclosed space, making the air—both inside and outside your body—more breathable.

Diffusing is useful for clearing the air, healing upper respiratory issues when you are sick, setting a mood, and/or preparing for sleep. It is a gentle application. That being said, diffused oils don't stay in the air long; a 2008 study showed that when lavender, eucalyptus, and tea tree oils were diffused, their antimicrobial effect improved air quality for about an hour but needed to be replenished after that. When you diffuse any oil, it's recommended that you only diffuse it for thirty minutes to an hour and then take an hour-long break before diffusing again. Studies indicate that leaving a diffuser on for longer than an hour diminishes its benefits. Many diffusers are equipped with timers, but you can also purchase an inexpensive timer at a local hardware store.

Currently, scientists are exploring how diffused essential oils can detoxify and improve indoor air quality. As the studies continue, one thing is clear: essential oils are useful for their antimicrobial, antibacterial effect in places where people are sick or are, by necessity, in close proximity to one another, like schools, airplanes, mass transit, and of course your home. Just be aware that when you diffuse an essential oil in a common area, you are affecting those around you as well.

INGESTING ESSENTIAL OILS: DON'T DO IT

Dear reader, I'm afraid I'm going to recommend you do not ingest essential oils. Although ingesting essential oils can be done safely under the supervision of a qualified aromatherapist, any professional would also check with your physician first to make sure doing so is okay for you. There is a lot written on the Internet about ingesting essential oils, but what many people don't know is that consuming essential oils can cause gastritis and even more serious reactions.

Please don't put peppermint oil into the water you drink, which can cause esophageal reflux. Since essential oils don't dissolve in water, drops of peppermint (or any essential oil) can lodge on the delicate mucous membranes in your digestive tract. Instead, have an occasional natural mint or use an essential oil toothpick. And you can get a healthy dose of essential oils just by twisting a couple of slices of an *organic* citrus fruit into a glass of filtered water or organic tea. Less is always more when you use essential oils wisely.

Applying

Applying essential oils externally, to the skin, is another way to create a significant internal effect within your body. Though absorption is less immediate than inhalation (it can take as long as twenty hours to absorb an essential oil applied topically) and the amount of microparticles less great (when you apply an essential oil topically you absorb anywhere from 5 to 20 percent of it through your skin, depending on the dilution of the oil), the effects of the oil are potent nonetheless. And topical application has advantages inhalation does not. For example, with topical application, you experience a time-release effect. If you apply a full-body oil (an essential oil diluted in a fatty oil) in the morning, it will help you sleep better that night, because the essential oil works on your nervous system throughout your day, long after the few hours of efficacy an inhaled or diffused oil has. And applying an essential oil product topically every day, over time, will affect your body in a deeper, more transformative way than the quick results of inhalation.

At the same time, while the oil is slowly absorbing, you are still inhaling its microparticles evaporating off your body. This aromatic cloud surrounds you like a protective aura, the microparticles flowing into your lungs and traveling to your brain. To take advantage of this dual action, essential oils applied to the face, neck, shoulders, and chest are most effective and are what I am recommending in this book.

When you apply essential oils topically, the microparticles mix with the natural oils of your skin and penetrate into the dermis below, which is why oils are so great for protecting the health of your skin (inside and out) as well as regenerating tissue. After penetrating the skin, the oils are absorbed through the lymphatic system and soft tissue underneath—your muscles, tendons, joints, and connective tissue—with numerous therapeutic results. Diuretic oils, like geranium, can move fluids trapped in the tissue (like the edema you can get from flying), while antispasmodic oils, like peppermint, relax your muscles. In addition, anti-inflammatory oils, like German chamomile, can reduce the swelling and redness associated with arthritis. Warming oils, such as rosemary, increase blood circulation by bringing more heat to an area, which opens up constricted blood vessels to promote healing.

Regardless of whether the essential oil is undiluted or diluted in a fatty oil for full-body application, the microparticles applied topically follow a similar path as the inhaled oil, traveling through the bloodstream to the endocrine system and organs, and are finally excreted through follicles in your skin or through your kidneys.

It's important to note both that when you apply oils topically, undiluted essential oils absorb faster than an essential oil mixed with another, fatty oil and that absorption happens more quickly when the skin is clean. But the most basic rule about applying essential oils is to target them right where you need them. If your sinuses are congested, put them at the opening of your nostrils. If your lower back is achy, apply them right there. The biggest benefit to targeting essential oils is that the journey to healing is shorter. Instead of having to work through your whole system, the microparticles are at their final destination from the moment you put your hand where it hurts.

Heating

Essential oils penetrate deeper when applied with heat, but never heat an oil over a flame because that will alter its chemical makeup. You *can* combine heat and essential oils through hydrotherapy, using water to heal. Simply apply the oils before taking a hot shower or add them to a warm bath.

"Water changes body temperature twenty-five times faster than air," says ASTECC-trained massage therapist Cherie Rodriguez and operations manager at Spa Montage in Laguna Beach, California. "When your body is heated up with hot water, your autonomic nervous system adjusts your body temperature through your circulation by dilating the blood vessels, opening the pores, relaxing the muscles, and allowing any excess fluids trapped in your legs and hips to flush out. Altogether you will relieve your stress and definitely sleep better if you do this at night."

During a long soak in the tub, you get hot and break a sweat, releasing toxins through your sweat ducts. Diuretic oils, like juniper, cypress, and geranium, can heighten this effect. The prolonged heat drives the oils deep into your muscles as you trigger a shift in your brain chemistry, called the "relaxation response" (which I'll explain more in chapter 4). Add some sleep oils to help release the sleep hormone melatonin and you will be down for the count.

If you don't like baths, try a shower. When you apply an essential oil blend to your chest and stand under the showerhead, the steam lifts the oil and makes it even more potent to inhale. The microparticles go deeper into your lungs as you breathe in the hot, essential-oil-laced air.

In fact, a shower may be the best place to absorb oils into congested lungs, especially when those oils are strong decongestants, like eucalyptus and pine. A shower may also be a way to detoxify and minimize allergies (which can be caused by a hypersensitive, toxic-laden immune system).

In chapter 2, I will discuss in detail how to use breathing exercises in the shower to reduce congestion and get rid of coughs, colds, allergies, and more.

My favorite method for combining heat and essential oils, however, is massage. With massage, the friction of the therapist's hands on your body creates heat, and the massage manipulates the soft tissue to drive the oils deeper in. Plus, with massage there's the proven psychological benefit of touch. And a good long massage gives you the chance to lie down and completely let go.

Finally, you can introduce heat by applying an oil topically to a targeted area and then covering that area with a hot compress or heating pad.

Getting Started with Essential Oils

By now, I hope you're excited about incorporating essential oils into your daily routine. Later in the book, I'll share details about how to buy and use oils to boost daily routines, address specific problems, and purify your home environment. For now, getting started is as easy as buying five basic, easy-to-find, affordable essential oils and one organic fatty oil you will use as a base for face, body, treatment, and massage oils.

Before I describe those five essential oils and the fatty oil, though, it's important to know that not all essential oils on the market are created equal. Harvested organic essential oils and/or wild-crafted oils (collected in the wild) that are steam-distilled are optimal for therapeutic use. These oils have a unique and complex structure that simply can't be replicated in a lab. However, the term "therapeutic" means something different for each company that supplies essential oils. It's no guarantee that a bottle labeled "natural" or "therapeutic" or "pure" will be an authentic substance.

Here's what you *should* look for on a bottle of essential oil:

- Its Latin botanical name (not just its common name)
- Its country of origin
- "Certified organic," "100% organic," or the USDA organic seal (the label or website will also include the name of the agency that certifies the oil, like OTCO or the European certifier "Ecocert"), or "wild-crafted" (picked in the wild)

Ideally, the essential oils you buy will have all this listed on their labels. When I create formulations at H. Gillerman Organics, I work only with 100% organic oils and try to source as many wild-crafted substances as I can. I'm able to do this by working with suppliers who have direct contact with their farmers, which creates a high level of accountability. These reputable farmers, manufacturers, and distributors work hard to create very high quality, efficacious oils that are available to us all.

Like I said, you can start exploring with just five essential oils and one organic fatty oil. Truly. There's really no need to go out and spend an entire paycheck on dozens of essential oils. I think it's easier, and thus more encouraging and empowering, to start with just a few essential oils that pack a big punch. The following five oils are what I recommend starting with. You can check out chapter 7 if you would like to read more about them. In my opinion, they are the most thoroughly researched, rejuvenating, cost-effective oils out there, so you can begin to reap the benefits by using these potent substances on a daily basis. For four of the oils I have suggested a second option, in case you prefer a different scent:

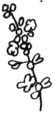

- *Lavender*

This all-purpose oil can be used as an antianxiety sleep aid, a muscle relaxant, a pain reliever, an antibacterial for wounds and burns, and a topical treatment for dry skin, eczema, and insect bites. It's also great for sachets and creating a "clean" scent throughout your home.

(You can substitute geranium oil if you prefer its sweeter, less herbaceous floral notes, and adjust my recipes if you find it too strong.)

• *Peppermint*

I call this the "new lavender" because it's definitely a contender in the essential oil popularity contest. Peppermint is a natural anti-inflammatory, working almost like liquid aspirin; it's one of the best for headaches. As an antiseptic, it can clear our breathing passages, treat the flu and colds, and help with digestive issues from simple stomachaches to irritable bowel syndrome (IBS) to morning sickness. If applied or inhaled an hour before bedtime, peppermint can aid sleep, but if you inhale it or use it during the day, it will help keep you awake. It's also a great detoxifier and room deodorizer—and best of all, a little goes a long way, so buying peppermint is very cost-effective. (Sorry, there is no substitute for peppermint!)

• *Tea tree*

Tested in hospitals as an effective treatment for antibiotic-resistant viruses (like MRSA), tea tree oil is a must for hygiene while traveling. With strong

antifungal properties, this oil helps alleviate respiratory infections, athlete's foot, burns, bites, infected wounds, and more. (If you're not crazy about the smell, feel free to substitute with niaouli or eucalyptus polybractea.)

• *Lemon*

This antiseptic oil is your go-to for cleaning; you can even use it straight on a sponge as you wipe down your kitchen counters. Lemon is an ideal oil to combine with others since it will increase the therapeutic effect and always add a bright note. A source for your daily antioxidant and vitamin C, this oil helps your body process toxins. (You can substitute grapefruit if you prefer its refreshing scent.)

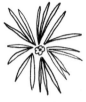

• *Cedarwood*

Cedarwood is a relaxing oil that helps hold scent on your body longer. For this reason, its scent is known as a base note, a term borrowed from perfumery. It's a great muscle relaxer. (You can substitute frankincense for cedarwood; it's a spicier, muskier, and more grounding oil than cedarwood, but it's more costly.)

• *The fatty oil: jojoba, golden or clear for unscented*

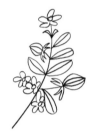

For safety and usability, essential oils need to be diluted in a base. Since essential oils don't dissolve in water, this base is usually a fatty oil: aromatherapists call this the "carrier oil." This fatty oil will serve as the ideal base for your face, body, treatment, and massage oils. A variety of rich emollient fatty oils, such as argan, rosehip seed, or even olive oil, can be combined with essential oils to create natural skin care products, but jojoba is best for both face and body. It doesn't clog pores and it closely matches the oil your own body produces (called sebum), so it absorbs well. It's appropriate for any skin type, including acne-prone skin. Because this oil has a longer shelf life than other fatty oils (in fact, it's a liquid wax that doesn't go rancid like seed and nut oils), I recommend always keeping an ample supply of it on hand.

That's it—all you need to get started. In chapter 4, you'll read about a wider range of oils you can add to your arsenal, and you can read more on these individual oils in chapter 7. In the meantime, discover in the chapters that follow the rituals using just these five essential oils. Whether you use these oils singly or combined into a blend is up to you. With just lavender, peppermint, tea tree, lemon, and cedarwood essential oils on hand, and a few simple formulas, you're ready to start exploring everyday self-care—and reaping its rewards. Enjoy!

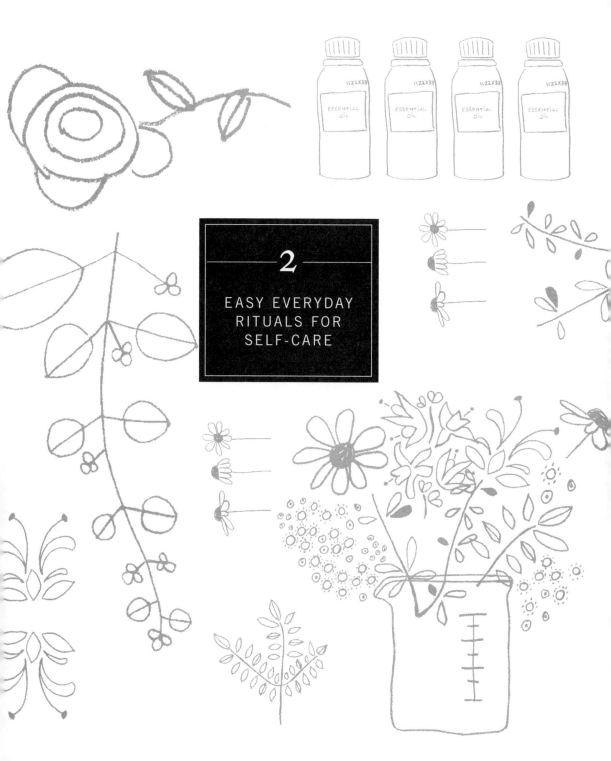

2

EASY EVERYDAY RITUALS FOR SELF-CARE

Back in 2008, when the economy was tumbling and no one was spending money on luxury natural beauty products, I was frantically trying to pitch my new line of high-quality organic essential oil blends to the founder of a chain of apothecary-style beauty boutiques, whom I'll call Mr. B. I knew I had only a few minutes, but I was surprised when he interrupted me during my very first sentence.

"What are these products and what do you do with them?" he asked. Immediately I thought, *They are the ultimate solution to stress!* Instead, I explained, "These are truly therapeutic, organic essential oil remedies, much more concentrated than a bath or body product. You apply them topically for pain or in the shower for deeper breathing, and you inhale them throughout the day to relax and focus." Mr. B responded, "They may be terrific problem solvers, but how often do most people use a remedy as compared to a body wash or shampoo? Not very often! And everyone knows what to do with their shampoo. How are you going to teach my customers what to do with essential oils?"

While Mr. B's response reflected a harsh reality, it put me on a course for my next task: to educate people on the true efficacy of essential oils. We use body care products *every day,* multiple times a day. Essential oils belong in this same category when it comes to personal care, front and center, used daily alongside our body washes and our makeup.

Rest assured, no matter how hectic your day may be, there is always time to take care of yourself and get back in touch with your body. And in this chapter I'll show you how easy it is to do that with essential oils. If you have already purchased your five oils, you are ready to start using them. If you want to use oils you have on hand, you can substitute. First, I will show you how easy it is to combine oils and dilute them yourself, and then I will go through a day of rituals you can try on for size. As you follow along, I will gently lead you toward a state of self-awareness and self-healing.

With essential oils, this can happen on many levels. So often, after I have taught a client an essential oil ritual, I hear comments like "Wow, after I applied that oil, I realized how much I was tensing my jaw" or "I didn't even know I was holding my breath." Unlike other basic self-care rituals, like brushing your teeth or washing your face, essential oils help you do something for your body *and* your mind, at the same time.

Dilution and Blending

First, let's talk about dilution and blending and key terms for the rituals that follow. A "100% essential oil" and a "100% essential oil blend" are straight, undiluted essential oils used either singly or in combination, called a "blend." "Massage oil," "face oil," "body oil," "treatment oil," and "perfume oil" are all made with essential oils mixed in a fatty oil base (see jojoba description). Mixing essential oils with a fatty oil is called "dilution." The Dilution Chart on pages 46–47 shows the different proportions for each type of oil. Essential oils are often diluted in other bases including alcohol (not a breathable base), liquid soap (washes off before fully absorbed), creams (includes additives), aloe vera (requires preservatives), and honey (just too sticky). For optimal therapeutic results, 100% essential oils in fatty oil dilutions are preferred.

Once you have made your blends and dilutions, you'll use the 100% blends for inhalations, massage oils for receiving or giving massages, face oils for nurturing skin care, body oils for all-over moisture and time-released absorption, treatment oils to target specific problems and sore areas, and perfume oils for your personal, mood-boosting aroma.

DILUTION CHART

Equivalents: 1oz. = 29.57 mL	30 drops = 1 mL	5 mL = 1 tsp.	15 mL = 1 tbsp.	1 oz. = 2 tbsp.	2 oz. = ¼ cup	4 oz. = ½ cup
Type of Product and Usage	% of essential oil to use a dilution of this specific type of product	Amount of EO to add to 5-mL European dropper	Amount of EO to add to 10-mL European dropper OR roll-on	Amount of EO to add to 1 oz. Boston round bottle	Amount of EO to add to 2-oz. Boston round bottle	Amount of EO to add to 4-oz. Boston round bottle
Massage Oil: for giving or receiving a single application for full body massage.	2%	3 drops	6 drops	18 drops	36 drops or ¼ tsp. approximately	72 drops or ½ tsp.
Body Oil: for full body application up to 2 times a day; if oil is gentle on skin use the full 5% or as desired	2–5%	not the right bottle for this product	6–15 drops in roll-on bottle	18–45 drops	36–90 drops or ¼–½ tsp. + 30 drops	½–1¼ tsp.
Treatment Oil: for targeted application on a limited area up to 3 times a day	15%	23 drops	45 drops	134 drops or a little less than 1 tsp.	2 scant tsp.	1 tbsp. + ½
Face Oil: to apply on damp skin, face, and neck area, as often as needed; use smaller percentage for sensitive skin or if new to essential oils in skin care	1–2%	2–3 drops	4–6 drops	9–18 drops	18–36 drops or ⅛–¼ tsp. approximately	36–72 drops or ¼–½ tsp.
Perfume Oil: to anoint pulse points up to 3 times a day	15–25%	23–52 drops	46–100 drops in roll-on bottle	Only make in small batches so that you can change your blend every 4–6 weeks		
Pregnancy Body Oil: apply on target area or full body; also use for elderly or sick on a target area	1%	2 drops	4 drops	9 drops	18 drops	36 drops or ¼ tsp.
Young Kids Body Oil: for children 1 to 5 years, on target area or have them inhale; for 1-year-olds, use less than 1%	1%	1 drop	2 drops	9 drops	18 drops	36 drops or ¼ tsp.
Kids Body Oil: for children 6 to 12 years	2%	3 drops	6 drops	18 drops	36 drops or ¼ tsp.	72 drops or ½ tsp.

For sensitive skin	Use hydrosols, which are ideal facial toners that balance pH and tighten pores.
For babies 0–12 months	Don't use essential oils on or near babies, but hydrosols are gentle enough to spray in the child's room.
For children 1–5 years	Use a young kids body oil on the chest, or apply the oil first to the back or chest before a bath. For inhalation, hold an oil-dampened tissue away from the child's nose.
For children 6–12 years	Use the body oil for 1- to 5-year-old children, but use the adult treatment oil formula to treat cuts and wounds with antiseptic oils (like lemon) and healing oils (like lavender and helichrysum).
For teenagers	Use the adult formulas topically and for inhalation (teenagers need the benefits!).
For the elderly	Dilute as per the pregnancy oil and apply it on the arms, hands, and feet. If the person is responding, you can also apply it to the neck, shoulders, and trunk.
For those who are seriously ill or in hospice care	Use less and dilute as per the pregnancy oil. If the patient is taking medications, consult their doctor first for any drug interactions (for example, grapefruit speeds up drug absorption, which changes the dosage; other essential oils can interact with chemotherapy). Essential oils do not work well with homeopathic formulations.
For pets	Though animals respond very well to essential oils, they are also very sensitive to smell (for example, there is a punishing collar that sprays dogs with citronella every time the dog barks). Avoid topical application if you can. When you want to calm and soothe, have the pet inhale from the bottle or put essential oils on a rag and put the rag in their bed or in front of their nose. If your dog or cat likes the oil, they may move their nose closer or turn their head slightly to the side (to lessen its intensity). If your pet doesn't like the oil, they will abruptly turn their heads away. For a pest repellent, dilute essential oils in a hydrosol and spray the mixture directly on the fur, or dilute essential oils in a fatty oil using the formula for a 1- to 5-year-old child. Put ¼ teaspoon in your palms, rub your palms together to mix the oil, and then wipe your hands over your pet's back, avoiding the pet's face and chin or anywhere they can lick it off. Keep this dilution away from cats.
How to blend in your palms on the fly	To save time when you don't have a premixed blend on hand, there is an easy method for blending a massage or body oil in your hands. Put 3 to 5 drops of essential oils in your palm first, then add about ½ teaspoon of the fatty oil (our palms can't hold much more) and rub the oils together in your palms before spreading them.

Once you set up your materials, making blends is a snap—and a relaxing experience in its own right. All you need to do is assemble your oils, storage bottles (a few 1-, 2-, and 4-ounce Boston rounds and 5- and 15-milliliter European droppers; for how to purchase these, see the resources section), and adhesive labels, grab a glass to mix the oils in, and find a comfortable, well-ventilated place to work. Have a notepad and a glass of water on hand too, which you must drink up while blending. (When you work with essential oils, you need to ensure you are hydrated to help the oils do their cleansing action and move through your system properly).

I recommend blending your essential oils first to get your desired aroma before diluting. Combine them in a wineglass or brandy snifter. These goblets are designed for swirling, which is the correct technique for blending essential oils. (The shape of a wineglass or brandy snifter is perfect for blending, because the tapered bell of the glass helps funnel the scent to your nose and gives you a stronger, truer impression of the scent than if you were to smell it straight from a bottle.) Adjust the blends as you wish, one drop at a time, smelling the blend fully after each addition and taking notes on any changes you make so that you can always make more!

For dilutions, you'll blend your primary oils in the same way, then transfer them into an applicator bottle, add your jojoba oil base, and tip the bottle up and down until fully mixed. (If you are making a large amount of finished dilutions [such as 8 ounces], use a small silicone spatula to fully mix everything before transferring it into your storage bottle.) Attach a label with its name and date, and store it away from light and heat. And use it often!

Here are some basic recipes for blends, using your starter set of five essential oils plus your jojoba oil (and a few optional extras). You can use these recipes any time a ritual in this chapter calls for a massage or body oil. There are also starter blends for face, treatment, and perfume oils and a diffuser blend.

Massage Oil

Blend: 30 drops lavender or geranium + 4 drops peppermint + ¼ teaspoon cedarwood or frankincense

Dilute: Transfer your essential oil blend into a 4-ounce Boston round bottle, add jojoba to fill (approximately ½ cup), and tip it upside down and then right-side up repeatedly—do not shake the bottle—and then label it. This massage oil is more therapeutic when applied during a massage or applied as a body oil, after a shower, prior to your session.

Benefits: Stimulates blood circulation, eases pain, relaxes the mind and body, and brings a glow to the skin.

Body Oil

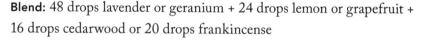

Blend: 48 drops lavender or geranium + 24 drops lemon or grapefruit + 16 drops cedarwood or 20 drops frankincense

Dilute: Put your essential oil blend in a 2-ounce Boston round bottle, add jojoba to fill (approximately ¼ cup), and tip it upside down and then right-side up repeatedly—do not shake the bottle—and then label it. Do a full-body application after a shower or bath or before traveling.

Benefits: Smoothes and slims the body and uplifts mood.

Treatment Oil

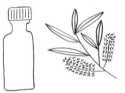

Blend: 18 drops tea tree or eucalyptus (or 9 drops of each) + 90 drops lavender + 18 drops cedarwood or frankincense. For a pain-relief version, add 3 drops peppermint + 2 drops helichrysum + 3 drops birch

Dilute: Put your essential oil blend in a 1-ounce Boston round bottle, add jojoba to fill (approximately 2 tablespoons), and tip it upside down and then right-side up repeatedly—do not shake the bottle—and then label it. For the pain-relief version, apply it by hand or roll it on the chest and shoulders. Put a few drops at the opening of each nostril for congestion.

Benefits: Decongests, deepens breathing, soothes when a person is feeling under the weather, and keeps muscles healthy. The pain-relief version is also slimming.

Basic Face Oil

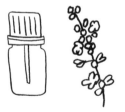

Blend and dilute: Add 5 drops lavender, geranium, or frankincense to 15-milliliter European dropper, add jojoba to fill (approximately 1 tablespoon), and tip it upside down and then right-side up repeatedly—do not shake the bottle—and then label it. Use 4 to 8 drops per application on clean damp skin.

Benefits: Sinks into the skin deeply without leaving it oily, to nurture, balance, regenerate, and moisturize, for all skin types.

Perfume Oil

Blend: 2 drops lavender or geranium + ½ teaspoon lemon + 2 drops ylang-ylang + 1 drop jasmine

Dilute: Put the essential oil blend into a 15-milliliter European dropper bottle, add jojoba to fill (approximately 1 tablespoon), and tip it upside down and then right-side up repeatedly—do not shake the bottle—and then label it. Anoint a drop on perfume points two or three times a day.

Benefits: A happy scent to refresh the mind while it attracts.

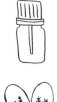

Diffuser Oil

Blend: Mix ¾ teaspoon eucalyptus or tea tree + 1½ teaspoons lemon or grapefruit in a 15-milliliter European dropper, and tip it up and down to blend.

Dilute: Add 5 to 10 drops of the essential oil blend directly into a diffuser filled with water to the fill line. Set your diffuser to intermittent setting.

Benefits: Cleans the air, boosts immunity, and wakes you up.

Basic Breathing

Since inhaling an essential oil is the *fastest* way to experience essential oil therapeutics, this is where to begin. The following simple exercise shows you how to properly inhale an essential oil, for the deepest intake of the microparticles, and it's the foundation for using essential oils every day. Once you've mastered this step, all the other benefits will follow.

SLOW BREATHING INHALATIONS

1. Select any 100% essential oil or oil blend.

2. Hold the bottle up to your nose and take a quick sniff.

3. Take note of any immediate association with this smell. The connection you make doesn't even have to be positive. "It smells like medicine" or "It smells like peanut butter" are equally valid. Remember the story of peppermint smelling like a candy that your grandmother gave you—any association you make is just your mind scrambling to identify the odor by connecting it with something you've smelled before.

4. For a deeper inhalation, sit comfortably in a chair, leaning back and relaxing your shoulders, and put 2 or 3 drops of the oil on a tissue or cotton ball. Exhale your next breath quietly and completely. Always completely exhale first before breathing in. After all, you don't go to a gas station with a full tank; you go when your tank is almost empty and ready to fill up. The same is true with breathing. If you start with an exhale, emptying out your lungs, your next breath will be a full tank of air—minimum effort for maximum oxygen. This will make you feel energized and at ease all at once.

5. As you finish your exhale, hold the tissue up to your nose, and this time very slowly and silently breathe the oil in. If you hear yourself making a sniffing sound, try to relax your nostrils (the sniffing sound is an indication you may be tightening and narrowing your breathing passages, making it harder to take in the full body of the aroma). It can be helpful to imagine that you are sipping in the oil through your nose, as if it were a straw, in one long inhale.

6. Exhale and inhale slowly again, waving the tissue back and forth below each of your nostrils, one side at a time. Smelling is three-dimensional, so each nostril "sees" the aroma a little differently. Feel free to experiment with how different the oil smells when you block one nostril.

7. Exhale and inhale slowly once more without blocking off your nostrils, and note how different the aroma is from when you first sniffed it. Try to feel the oil entering your body through your breathing passages. You may even feel the oil going to specific parts of your body. (For example, you may feel pine moving into your chest or eucalyptus traveling up into your sinus passages or sandalwood going way down to the bottom of your ribs where your primary breathing muscle, the diaphragm, is located.)

8. Continue to slowly exhale and inhale. Now try to relax your abdominals a bit so that your breathing gets even deeper. You can even put a hand on your belly to feel when you are letting your muscles ease up. Pay attention to your belly, which should be moving while you breathe: flattening when you exhale and relaxing when you inhale. Don't worry about keeping your core muscles taut when doing this breathing exercise.

A powerful alternative to breathing in your oils from a tissue or cotton ball is to breathe them in from your palms. Here's how: Put a drop or two of any single oil or oil blend in the center of one palm. Heat up the oil by rubbing your palms together quickly. Exhale completely and then cup your hands over your face for your inhalations. If the oil feels too strong, move your hands farther away. If you are tensing your shoulders, put your elbows on a desk or table for support while breathing in the oil.

After this exercise, you should be feeling the oils working on your psyche and relaxing your body. This simple technique is a go-to method for adjusting your mood, clearing your sinuses, alleviating tension, and sleeping better. Mastering the fine art of exhaling to slowly breathe in an essential oil is an extremely useful skill, not only in the moment, to help you breathe more deeply, but also for your whole life!

You Only Have to Make Time for One Ritual

There are so many options for incorporating healing essential oils into daily life, choosing where to start can seem overwhelming. But here's the thing: it doesn't matter which specific ritual you choose, I promise, because using the oil is what really matters. You can start by exploring some of the following rituals using oils you already own, the five oils from chapter 1, or the blends from this chapter. Some mornings your favorite oil or oil blend will feel right, but the next day it might not. Don't worry. Your body is just talking to you and telling you what it needs. You can't go wrong, just as long as you have the basic oils that are right for you.

You can try doing one ritual a day or up to one ritual per time of day (like during the morning, at work, or in the evening). Remember, when it comes to essential oils—nature's most concentrated medicine—less is more. (You'll see this repeated throughout the book, because it bears repeating.) Let each ritual you practice bring your thoughts and focus back to yourself, your mind, and your body. Maybe your body needs to get up and stretch, or to yawn and breathe more deeply. Maybe your body needs a quick nap, the oldest trick in the book for staying healthy and alert. Maybe your mind needs a few minutes of calm and quiet. Using essential oils every day brings the space and clarity needed for self-awareness and true self-care.

In the Morning: Starting Your Day with Essential Oils

First thing in the morning is one of the best times to use essential oils because you can combine slow breathing inhalation, drawing fresh oxygen and essential oils into your lungs and brain, with all-day absorption. Here's how to get this ideal double dosage: apply a few drops of a single oil or oil blend to your temples, neck, shoulders, or chest, where your skin is thinnest and closest to your all-important nose, and include a few slow breathing inhalations from your fingertips after you apply. To absorb even more of the plants' healing essences, apply essentials oils to clean, warm skin, like after your shower or bath. To get off on the right foot, always start your morning with the oils, or oil blends, that put you in a good mood right away. These could be one of your five starter oils or starter oil blends—the bright refreshing citrus oils, a stimulating spice, a beautiful flower blend, or a meditative oil—whatever works for you.

> Always drink a glass of water when you first wake up to help cleanse from within! Hydrating helps your liver clear toxins and your body and mind complete the process of "rest and digest" that sleep provides.

UPON WAKING (WHILE STILL IN BED)

Anoint your sinus-clearing facial acupoints by placing 1 small drop of your chosen wake-up oil or oil blend (lavender, tea tree, and/or lemon) on the tip of each index finger and setting your fingertips beside the bridge of your nose. You might even feel little pockets that you can rest your fingers in—these are called acupoints. If you press lightly into your face and then, with a slight twist of your hands, separate your fingers slightly, you will feel your nasal passages opening. Repeat slow breathing inhalations five or six times. This will set your mood and deepen your breathing for the whole day.

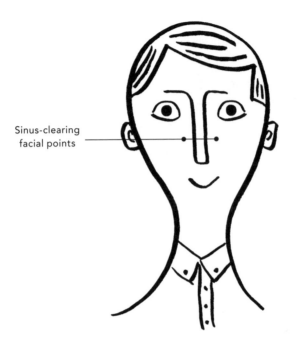

Sinus-clearing
facial points

HOW TO PRACTICE YOGA IN BED

This works very well after your sinus-clearing Upon Waking ritual. After
a rough night of not sleeping, or even after I've gotten a luscious nine
hours, I sometimes have trouble getting going in the morning. But
I've adapted a great yoga sequence I learned at the YinOva Center
to wake me up, which always gets me breathing, moving, and feeling
ready to go, physically and mentally! And best of all, there's no need
to change clothes, use a mat, or find enough space on the floor.

1. *Alternate nostril breathing:* Place a drop of a decongesting 100%
essential oil (use tea tree, eucalyptus, or niaouli) under your nostrils.

Keeping your eyes closed, close your right nostril with your thumb and exhale through your left nostril; then close your left nostril with an index finger and slowly inhale through your right nostril. Repeat the sequence two times, then reverse: close your left nostril and exhale through your right nostril; then close your right nostril and inhale through your left nostril. Also repeat this sequence two times. Keep your breathing slow and easy as you continue.

2. *Mini Cobra:* Roll over onto your belly with your hands by your shoulders and push your hands down into the mattress to lift your shoulders, then your chest. Finally, lift your head into a mini back bend (baby Cobra position).

3. *Savasana:* Release out of the Cobra and roll over onto your back and stretch your whole body in a big X.

4. *Back stretch:* Bend one knee toward your chest. Holding on to your shin or the top of your knee, gently guide the knee close to your chest to stretch your back. Extend the leg and repeat this with your other knee. This should be a very easy stretch. If your back feels supertight, instead bend both knees, put your palms on the tops of the knees, and slowly rotate the knees to warm up your lower back.

5. *Twist:* Add in your favorite twist that feels great and opens up your body, such as crossing one knee or both knees over your body.

6. *Cross-legged position:* Slowly roll onto your side and sit up in a cross-legged position. Stretch your neck by tipping your chin down toward your collarbone.

7. *Chair pose:* Swing your legs over the side of the bed and stand up as if you are coming out of a squat. Optional: Finish with a Downward-Facing Dog pose with your hands on the edge of the bed.

After some simple yoga in bed, you will be good to go!

WHILE YAWNING

Smooth from cheekbone to jawline a face-friendly, relaxing essential oil dilution (use the basic face oil recipe on page 50). Then separate your back molars as if you were holding a blueberry between your teeth—if you tense your jaw muscles, you will squish it. Next, pull your tongue off the roof of your mouth and drag the heels of your hands from the start of your cheekbones, in front of your ears, down and forward along the edge of your jawline three times.

Now try fake yawning three or four times. Make the yawns as big as possible. Fake yawns often give way to the real thing, so let 'er rip. There is nothing better for a tight jaw than yawning. Yawning even cleanses your tear ducts and brightens your eyes. Think of it as a stretch for your breath.

BEFORE YOU STEP INTO THE SHOWER

Dry-brush the back of your neck, tops of your shoulders, and lower back with a loofah, brush, or puff, then smooth into these muscles a relaxing essential oil dilution (use the treatment oil recipe on page 50). Step into the shower and let the pressure and heat of the water hitting your body pound into these tight areas. Stay tension- and/or pain-free all day by remembering this moment and consciously relaxing these areas again.

IN THE HEAT OF THE SHOWER

Put 2 drops of 100% essential oil (tea tree, niaouli, or eucalyptus) at the opening of each nostril or along your collarbone. You may have a favorite decongesting blend that will work perfectly here, or check out the Breathing program in chapter 4 for some suggestions. Stand facing the showerhead and let the steam fill your lungs as you do five slow breathing inhalations. To deepen the effect, exhale with a whispered *ah* sound, which also decongests the vocal cords.

AFTER YOUR SHOWER

When your skin is freshly exfoliated and your pores are open, your skin is prepped for optimal absorption. After toweling yourself dry, apply an essential oil dilution all over your entire body (use the body oil recipe on page 49). Remember, less is more: you don't have to pour on the oil. Pour ½ teaspoon into your palm, rub your hands together, and smooth the oil over one body part at a time—your legs, arms, hips, chest, and abdomen.

Another option after a shower is to apply 1 drop of 100% essential oil, or 2 drops diluted in a little jojoba oil in your palm for sensitive skin (use lavender, tea tree, cedarwood, and/or frankincense), to each armpit before you apply deodorant (or in lieu of deodorant). This will send healing oils into your lymphatic system as well. You can also drop these same oils between your toes as a deodorant for your feet. But don't bother applying oil to the soles of your feet because this is *not* an absorbing area.

WHILE GETTING DRESSED

Because essential oils are not oily like olive or nut oils (fatty oils), you can drop clear ones, such as eucalyptus, lavender, or tea tree, onto your clothes. Tap a few drops of any clear-colored 100% essential oil onto a lapel or neckline near your face. This is a great way to hold the scent near your nose for extended, passive inhalation. It works best on natural-fiber fabrics, since the fibers have spaces between them, which become tiny vessels for the oils. Note: Avoid clothes that would show a water stain, like silk.

If you prefer, you can buy essential oil patches for passive inhalation, but they are not optimal because the oils aren't fresh.

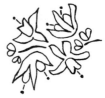

At Work: Keeping Calm and Focused with Essential Oils

To save you time and get instant relief, inhaling essential oils will be your go-to method throughout your workday. If you're really pressed for time and can't fit in one of these daytime rituals, just apply some oils to your neck, your throat, the tops of your shoulders, and your chest, and let the inhalation begin!

FOR A QUICK DESK BREAK

Sit back in your chair, resting your elbows on the chair arms. Place a drop of a single 100% essential oil (lavender, peppermint, and/or lemon) into your palms and rub them together. Cup your palms over your face, and do six slow breathing inhalations with your eyes closed.

TO FRESHEN UP YOUR OFFICE

Keep a wineglass or brandy snifter on your desk and tap a few droplets of your favorite 100% single essential oil or oil blend into the glass. (While they sit on your desk, the oils in them evaporate gradually, like a passive diffuser.) Your daytime blend can be whatever puts you in a good mood without slowing you down (use lemon, peppermint, or lavender, or see chapter 4 for ideas on creating the perfect daytime blend for you). If you need a slow breathing inhalations break, just breathe in from the glass.

FOR DAYTIME MEDITATION

Put a drop of 100% essential oil (use frankincense or cedarwood, or for sensitive skin use the perfume oil recipe) on the tip of each index finger. Anoint key acupoints on your face, such as your temples, the inside edges of your eyebrows, and in front of your ears (this is a jaw tension release point). Place your fingertips lightly on each point, not massaging but gently resting there. After five seconds, make very slow, tiny circles to soothe the nervous system. To prolong this mindful moment, sit back, rest the backs of your hands in your lap, and practice slow breathing inhalations, making sure you completely exhale first and watching the movement of your body as the breaths travel in and out. Reapply the oil before the inhalations if needed.

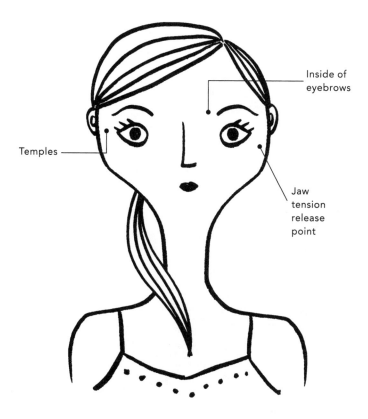

Inside of eyebrows

Temples

Jaw tension release point

TO WAKE UP AND FOCUS

Place a drop of a decongesting 100% essential oil (use tea tree, eucalyptus, or niaouli) at the opening of each nostril to clear your breathing passages. Then anoint your sinus-clearing facial acupoints to increase alertness. Put a few drops of a stimulating blend on the back of your neck.

After, sit at the front edge of your chair, clasp your hands together, and cradle the back of your head in your hands. Stretch your neck and your spine by lifting the back of your head with your hands. You will find you are now sitting quite straight but not stiffly, and your abdominal muscles will be tighter and your breathing easier. Use the oils as needed to remind you to breathe and sit well.

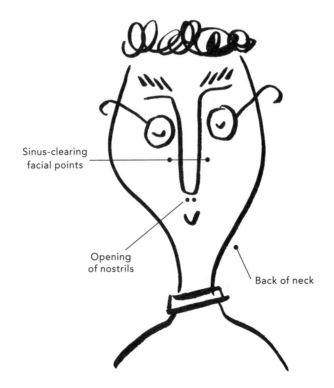

Sinus-clearing facial points

Opening of nostrils

Back of neck

FOR A TENSION BREAK

On each side of your neck, your shoulders, and your lower back, smooth ¼ teaspoon of a muscle-relaxing dilution oil (use the treatment oil recipe on page 50). Push your chair back from your desk. Sit with your arms folded genie-style and rest them on the front edge of your desk. Elongate your spine as you bend forward to rest your forehead heavily on your forearms. Focus on relaxing your neck as you rest.

HOW TO SIT FOR LONG PERIODS, IF YOU MUST, TO STAY FOCUSED AND PAIN-FREE

I can't tell you how many people I've taught to do this, and how much it helps them to avoid fatigue and back pain while it also aids digestion, facilitates deep breathing, and keeps the mind alert. In short, it's your best option if you can't stand. Once you learn how to sit correctly, it will take a second for your body to adjust. Make sure you don't force anything. Every time I do this, I say to myself, "Hey, you, why didn't you do this sooner? This is so much better." I guarantee, once you begin practicing this posture every day, your body will loosen up without effort. Yay!!!

1. Take your hands off your keyboard and push away from your desk. Adjust the seat of your chair so your hips are above the level of your knees—this will keep your hip muscles from cramping.

2. To adjust your body position, first move to the front edge of your chair, with your feet on the ground, feeling your sitting bones right underneath your ears. Clasp your hands behind your back and squeeeeeeeze your shoulders together to get rid of the rounding in

your upper back. Lift your chest if you need to feel more of a stretch. Bring your chin to your chest to stretch the back of your neck.

3. Release your hands and move your keyboard closer to you so that you can touch the keys while keeping your elbows alongside your torso and bent at a ninety-degree angle. This may feel much lower and closer than you would think.

4. Adjust your screen so that you are looking slightly down (especially if you are wearing progressive lenses), but beware: most of us sit with our heads pushing toward the screen. Please don't do this. It hurts!

5. Add an essential oil lift: Apply an essential oil dilution (use the treatment oil, pain-relief version, on page 50) to your neck and shoulders, clasps your hands, and cradle the back of your neck, right underneath the base of your skull, lifting to stretch your neck and straighten your spine. Stretch your elbows farther apart to open and lift your chest. Ahhh, now you can breathe. If your back gets tired, move your hips all the way back in your chair, put a cushion or folded-up towel behind your upper or lower back, whichever feels more comfortable, and lean your whole back against the chair. This should feel fantastic.

During Exercise: Essential Oils to Stay Flexible and Pain-Free Through Your Workout

Diluted essential oils work over time, with a time-release effect. Whether you apply your oils before your workout (or yoga) or after, you will be targeting right where you need them. To pretreat an injury on the mend, warm up your stiff zone, or get a deeper stretch, the oils will speed up the action. Plus, you will become more sensitive to what your body needs throughout your workout because your body feels more responsive.

BEFORE YOUR WORKOUT

Locate the areas or muscles that are limiting your fullest range of movement, for example, a stiff ankle, a stiff lower back, or a painful neck. Smooth over the area a workout oil blend (use the treatment oil, the pain-relief version, on page 50, if needed). Rub the area to create friction and heat. Gently mobilize the tight or painful area without pushing your limit or holding your breath.

AFTER YOUR WORKOUT

Target an area by applying your workout oil to any muscle that feels fatigued or stiff from the workout. Rub the area to create a little friction and heat for deeper penetration. To stretch, wait for five exhales on each stretch to give your body time to adjust and let go. At home you can follow with a hot compress or heating pad on the area before going to bed. Repeat the sequence in the morning.

Do not stretch a muscle in spasm; just rest and the oils will do the work for you.

TO TARGET AN INJURY

Follow the directions for "After Your Workout" (even if you aren't working out), using the treatment oil dilution, the pain-relief version, on page 50, but do *not* rub or stretch a newly injured area. If it is an older injury, apply a hot compress or heating pad and add some friction to the area by rubbing it. Apply oils twice a day for pain and injuries (see chapter 7 for more detail).

BEFORE YOUR YOGA PRACTICE

To get your breathing working for you in your practice, start with a drop of a decongesting 100% essential oil (use eucalyptus, niaouli, or tea tree) at the opening of each nostril.

HOW TO GET A MINI WORKOUT ANYTIME

Fred DeVito, an exercise innovator, wellness expert (what a perfect combo), and co-creator of the Core Fusion program, truly knows the value of essential oils for a healthy, mindful, and productive fitness lifestyle. He uses essential oils to help boost awareness of where his body is in the moment and of old injuries. He shared this simple yet perfect sequence with me so that I could share it with you. He calls it the Trunk Rotation and Side Bend exercise.

1. Apply the treatment oil dilution (use the pain-relief version on page 50, if needed) to your lower back and hips.

2. Stand with your feet slightly wider than your hips, with your arms relaxed at your sides, and take three deep breaths.

3. Raise your arms at your sides as high as your shoulders and twist your trunk to the right as you look over your right shoulder.

4. As you twist to the right, lift your left heel slightly. Return to facing forward, then repeat the movement toward the left, raising your right heel slightly. Repeat the sequence on each side five times.

5. Lower your arms and face forward, standing still.

6. Raise your right arm above your shoulder and slide your left arm down your left side as you side-bend to the left. Repeat the same movement on the opposite side. Repeat the bends five times on each side.

You'll notice this gets your breathing going with a bonus of abdominal toning and a balance challenge for your use 'em or lose 'em muscles. To test my balance more, I like to see how far I can twist with both heels lifted and then peek at the hand behind me. The best time to do this exercise is in the morning, but feel free to practice it any time you need to get up and stretch. And for the all-time quickest workout at your desk, do squats in and out of your chair, keeping your back straight and your neck long.

So you see, you always have time to get your blood moving, especially with some circulation-pumping essential oils on your ankles, feet, and calves (use the pain-relief version of the treatment oil on page 50 for this effect).

At Night: Essential Oils to Shift Gears, Slow Down, and Sleep

Here's when having a routine really pays off. By incorporating an essential oil ritual into your nightly routine, you signal your brain that your workday is done.

WHEN YOU ARRIVE HOME

Create a quick environmental change by diffusing a single 100% essential oil or oil blend (use lavender, lemon, frankincense, and/or cedarwood) or by applying a few drops of a 100% clear oil (such as lavender) to a pillow or, after changing into comfortable clothing, to the fabric of what you're wearing.

TO SWITCH GEARS

Smooth a relaxing face oil dilution (use the face oil recipe on page 50) from cheekbone to chin with the heel of your hand, moving down and then forward along the line of your jaw. Massage your temples gently with the same diluted oil.

TO REENERGIZE BEFORE A NIGHT OUT

Tap a few drops of a stimulating 100% essential oil (like peppermint) on the back of your neck. Lightly dry-brush your legs and apply a stimulating oil dilution (use the treatment oil recipe, pain-relief version, on page 50) to the tops of your feet, ankles, and calves with upward strokes for a spring in your step.

AFTER YOUR CLEANSING ROUTINE

On your neck and shoulders, smooth a presleep oil dilution (use 2 drops of the perfume oil recipe on page 51), using the opposite hand when applying the oil to each shoulder (e.g., apply the oil to your right shoulder with your left hand).

FOR EXTRA RELAXATION BEFORE BED

Try these techniques if you need help relaxing or your body feels tense. Lie on your back in bed with a heating pad under your neck or your lower back and pillows under your knees and calves. After a few minutes, your back and neck should feel looser. If you still can't relax, focus on easing neck tension: Clasp your hands behind your head and lift your head until your chin touches your chest. Imagine that your head is a heavy boulder so your arms do all the work, not your neck. Practice slow breathing inhalations to fully let go.

ANTISNORING PREPARATION

Fill a small glass bowl with boiling water and add 2 or 3 drops of a decongesting 100% essential oil (use tea tree, eucalyptus, or niaouli) on the top of the water. Close your eyes and hold your face over the bowl, breathing in the steam slowly until you feel your sinuses clearing. If your chest is congested, breathe in through your mouth. Then blow your nose (or cough) to clear breathing passages, and once you are in bed, practice slow breathing inhalations to fall asleep silently.

IN BED

Once in bed, prep a tissue or cotton ball with 2 or 3 drops of your chosen 100% essential oil sleep blend (lavender and frankincense). Turn off your lights if they are not already off. Exhale and then do at least ten slow breathing inhalations from the tissue or cotton ball. Stay mindful of your breath as you put the tissue aside and fall deeply asleep.

CREATE YOUR OWN AT-HOME SPA

If you are going for a massage, always shower before your treatment and follow the shower with a body oil application (use the massage oil recipe on page 49). Or if you are going for a pedicure, tap a few drops of oil on the top of each foot ahead of time—the foot soak at the salon will automatically turn into an aromatherapy footbath. But don't wait until you have the time and space to get to a spa; it's easy to achieve spalike pampering and relaxation without stepping out your door.

For a Pedicure

Place 1 drop of a single 100% essential oil or oil blend (use peppermint, cedarwood, and/or tea tree) on each toenail bed before soaking your feet. After soaking your feet, massage a diluted oil blend (use the massage oil recipe on page 49, body oil recipe on page 49, or treatment oil recipe on page 50) on your feet and up your calves before applying polish. Celebrity green nail stylist and "five-free formula" nail polish creator Jenna Hipp introduced me—and all her celebrity clients, like Lea Michele and Jessica Alba—to her innovative techniques on natural nail care with essential oils. She likes to start all her nail sessions with essential oils on the neck and shoulders to make the whole experience soothing and calming—and give her clients a way to feel more relaxed walking the red carpet.

For a Bath

Draw a warm but not too-hot bath. Step in and turn the spigot back on. Pour under the spigot about a ½ teaspoon diluted oil blend (use the massage oil recipe on page 49, body oil recipe on page 49, treatment oil recipe on page 50, or 2 drops of the perfume oil recipe on page 51) and encourage further dispersal by swishing the water and oil with your hands. Sitting in the bath, soak a washcloth in the water and gently rub it over your whole body, then place it on your chest. Lie back and relax every bone in your body. The heat and the oil work together to release melatonin, a hormone that helps you go to sleep. You will sleep like a baby after this bath.

For the Total Spa Experience

Before taking a shower, lightly brush your body all over in a circular motion using a dry brush or loofah. Make sure the water temperature of your shower is very warm before stepping in. Let the heat of the shower relax your muscles for a minute or two, then gradually adjust the water to a cooler setting and let it run over your scalp for a minute. Switch back to warm water for another minute and then finish with cold water. If it is cold outside, end on a last minute of warm water instead. Pat your body dry with a towel and apply to your full body a diluted oil blend. This method also releases the sleep hormone melatonin. You can do this ritual right before bed if you need help getting to sleep.

If you did get to a commercial spa, you can switch back and forth between the hot tub and the cold plunge—the ultimate spa ritual to prep you for the deepest, most relaxing massage.

I began doing this method as a child without even knowing it, walking down the beach on hot days, going from hot sun and sand into the cold ocean water and repeating that until I finally jumped in for a swim. It's exhilarating and ultimately relaxing.

Change Just One Habit and More Will Follow

I hope you're encouraged to try at least one of these rituals, if not more, after reading this chapter. If one of the rituals you try feels really good, it's okay to start by doing just that one each day.

Be sure to practice the slow breathing inhalations whenever you use oils. Just inhaling the oils properly is effective. And by doing inhalations or a ritual at the same time every day, you will more quickly instill using essential oils as a habit.

Studies indicate that the more we exercise our willpower, the stronger it becomes. As a dancer, I know how daunting learning a new routine can be.

Dancers have to quickly learn not only new steps but also forty-five-minute-long, complex sequences of those steps. On that first day of practice, it always seemed hard to believe that at some point soon the new choreography would become second nature to me. But with conscious, intentional practice, it always did. And the same will be true for you with essential oils. When you practice every day, even just one ritual, using essential oils soon will become as second nature to you as your unconscious habitual behaviors—but infinitely more rewarding. You'll find it's easier than you could have believed to take good care of yourself while using nature's most concentrated medicine.

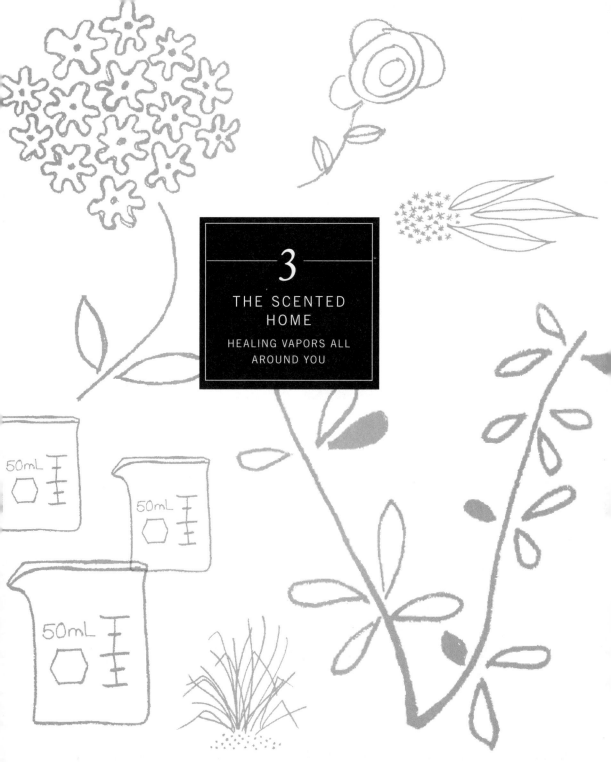

3

THE SCENTED HOME

HEALING VAPORS ALL AROUND YOU

Making my home in New York City for the past umpteen years has given me the best support system a creative person can ask for. My colleagues and I form a tight-knit group of people who care passionately about wellness and offer one another daily support. We search assiduously for the best benefits alternative and holistic methods can offer—and that's just what we get. I feel extremely lucky to have experienced treatments from many world-renowned healers on the knockabout streets of Manhattan. But despite the city being a relatively healthy environment spiritually, it's *not* a great place to be a nose.

There are a million unmentionable odors in the air of Manhattan. Even though my life is all about smell and the body, I have to shut down my senses to withstand these ugly odors, just like my fellow New Yorkers. This became a serious problem when I had to finalize the formulas for my line of therapeutic, organic essential oil blends. I knew that living every day with repellent fumes in the air would prejudice my nose to choose oils that shouted their scents loudly and overpowered other smells in the environment, good or bad. My constant need for breathable air was coloring my choices, and I felt like I was losing track of the subtle grace that nature's most vibrant elixirs have.

To clear my palate, I left my long-term home in Manhattan and moved into a treetop garret by a lush park in Fort Greene, Brooklyn. Thanks to the very old and beautiful trees and shrubs, I finally found air nourished by photosynthesis and free-flowing currents—which is what oxygen is supposed to smell like! This environment provided a more neutral olfactory base, which I needed to create my blends. With cleaner air, I didn't have to shut down my senses anymore, and my nose could finish the job I had given it.

So, what about your environment? Is it olfactory neutral? Or is your home scented with candles and sprays? Are you constantly struggling to cover up an animal odor or smells you just don't like? Many of us try to block out bad odors with artificial fragrances, including synthetic perfumes. But this practice not only is harmful from a health perspective (since synthetics are chock-full of harmful ingredients) but can also dull your sense of smell long-term, just like the bad odors of Manhattan once threatened to dull mine. A much better way to scent and clear the air within your home or your office is with essential oils.

To get an impression of how your home really smells, take a big whiff the next time you walk in the door after being outside. Do you like what you smell? Or could nature's most potent elixir make your home more relaxing?

The Most Beautiful Way to Transform a Home

Organic essential oils are the most beautiful, healthy way to scent your living space and work environment. These substances are not only safe, pure, and truly natural but also transport you to times and places in your life where you experienced these scents in their natural habitat: a beach, a forest, a rose garden.

Essential oils can shift your state of mind on physiological and chemical levels. Once you begin using essential oils to scent and clean your home, everyone in your home benefits. Your plants will flourish and even your pets will notice the soothing vapors. And when you come in from the cold or a difficult commute and diffuse a favorite scent in your home, you will feel like there is no place else you would rather be.

Because essential oils are antiseptic, they neutralize the odor-causing germs and microbes that pollute the air in your home. The more you slowly and fully inhale air that contains an essential oil, the more its scent will remind you what healthy air should smell like. You will immediately feel the difference when you switch to breathable scents in the air, and over time, your senses will become more attuned to picking up any toxic or unhealthy fragrances. This may sound like a negative, but being conscious of harmful off-gases and potentially toxic or unhygienic odors in your environment will help you choose better products for your children to play with, for your pets to sleep on, and for you to use throughout your home. It will be easy for you to avoid plastic-smelling drapes or a slightly moldy antique rug. It's possible to cleanse your world just by using your nose once you train it to become more reliable and sensitive.

When you evaporate essential oils in your home, you release a mist of antimicrobial, antiviral, antibacterial, antifungal agents—and even some antihistamines—all of which are immune boosters that keep your home clean and healthy for all. Obviously, you can't control all the toxins in your environment, but converting to organic oils helps to ensure you are living in the ultimate healing home.

Whenever someone enters my home, they always remark on the scent. I always say, "It better smell good with all the oils I work with!" But the truth is that unless I am formulating a new blend of oils, I have no idea exactly what the guest in my home smells. It could be the oil I used that morning or the trash by my desk where I threw out some essential-oil-drenched paper towels after cleaning up lunch dishes. (You know you are living well when your trash smells good!)

But it's easy and simple to have a remarkably aromatic home. Once you place essential oils strategically throughout your house (and use essential oils as cleaning products), each room will have its own unique scent and environment. Though invisible aroma-decorating doesn't play well on a home-makeover TV show, I can tell you, as an industry insider, that top decorators always add scent to a room as a final flourish.

Ideally, once you learn how to incorporate different essential oils throughout your home, the specific scents you've chosen for each space in your home will create a unique sensory world that will keep you and your guests breathing deeply, feeling relaxed, and exhaling *ahhhh* . . .

But first, we should explore how and why our homes smell at all!

What Our Noses Know

Using your sense memory, recall a moment when you suddenly encountered an alarming smell—like an airplane taking in jet fuel exhaust fumes while waiting for takeoff, the smoke from someone's cigarette, or perhaps the exhaust from a diesel engine.

Do you remember trying not to breathe? When I ask my clients to remember a feeling like this, many even recall the feeling of their nasal passages narrowing to avoid breathing in the bad air. But what a lot of us don't realize is how much we shut down our sense of smell every day, all day long, as we adapt to the overload of artificial and toxic aromas all around us. And with a dulled olfactory awareness, it takes a strong odor to get our attention. Over time, it's easy for us to lose touch with what truly natural aromas smell like: the delicate, sweet scent of a field of wildflowers or the clean, woodsy smell from the bark of a cedar tree as it wafts through a slightly damp forest. Our noses get used to the onslaught of the artificial— and we become numb to our noses.

It is no wonder that many of us seek out very strong, synthetic odors for our personal space. When we look for a scent that will make our home feel comforting—creating a signature for our home, our mark—we work with our memories. We choose fragrance-laden laundry soap because the detergent has a "clean smell." We choose strong air fresheners and candles because their scent reminds us of a luxurious perfume. Our cars are loaded with beloved "new car smell" air fresheners to prolong the exhilarating moment of the purchase.

But what most of us don't realize is that these unregulated, chemist-engineered fragrances come with a steep price: tons and tons of toxins entering our bodies through our lungs. It may seem like a big (and more expensive) switch to move away from these familiar odors and instead scent your world with essential oils, but using natural fragrance is the healthier—and much less costly—choice by far.

BEWARE THE REED DIFFUSER!

What disturbs me the most when I enter a client's home is seeing a reed diffuser (or worse yet, multiple reed diffusers!), a type of air freshener in which "reeds"—wooden sticks coated in absorbent material—are inserted into a bottle or jar of synthetic fragrance. The reeds absorb and draw the chemical compound up from the bottle and disperse it into the air.

Here's why reed diffusers bother me so much: some room fragrance contains phthalates (pronounced *thal-ates*), which are linked to reproductive issues, hormonal disruption, diabetes, obesity, and thyroid irregularities, and the reed coating contains dipropylene glycol, an ingredient used in antifreeze that is toxic to children and animals. Do you really want to be in this environment?

Yet another great reason to replace all the chemical fragrances in your home with organic essential oils!

It's also worth mentioning that bad smells do more than just color our preferences for "good" smells. Toxic odors affect our breathing patterns, making each inhalation shorter and tighter. Unconsciously, the body is trying to limit the amount of toxins we inhale by breathing more shallowly. But if we breathe that way long enough, there will be an inadequate intake of oxygen with each breath, making our brain function fuzzy, which in turn can make us feel fatigued, anxious, and/or depressed.

For many people, making their daily living environments cleaner and healthier means changing habits. I often see offices with their windows sealed shut. This allows harmful air and the substances within it to recirculate. I witnessed the negative effects of an environment like this at my very first spa industry trade show. The show was set up in a huge convention hall that had recently put in new carpet—a prime offender when it comes to everyday objects that off-gas nasty chemicals. After just a day in this chemical-laden, fresh-air-free convention hall, attendees were flocking to my booth to get help for their runny noses, congestion, and allergic responses.

But it's not just commercial spaces. When my friends tell me that their son has asthma or that a spouse just can't shake his chest cold or that they need twenty-four-hour allergy medication every single day, I struggle to stay silent as I suspect the culprit is the cleaning products and chemicals used to make their homes smell "good."

Problematic Cleaning Products

The vast majority of cleaning products are made up of toxic chemicals and synthetic fragrances. Even the "organic" and "sustainable" product lines can contain laureth sulfates, artificial cleansing agents that are also known carcinogens. On websites like the Environmental Working Group's EWG .org, you can look up the products you're currently using in your home and learn about the health hazards of each ingredient. EWG.org and other green-living websites and blogs have great suggestions for toxin-free options to replace the chemicals you should definitely throw away (like, right now).

Or just use your nose! If you can't inhale a deep breath of what's in a bottle, don't use it.

It's important to remember that when you reach for a product with a clean, transparent design or an illustration of a plant or a flower on the label along with words like "natural" or "simple" or "basic," you could still be buying the *most* toxic product in the store. Many of these products not only are loaded with carcinogenic foaming agents but build their aroma on synthetic fragrances, *not* real herbs or essential oils. Often an essential oil is added to the ingredient list of a product so the manufacturer can claim the product is "natural," when in fact the quantity of essential oil used in the product is negligible. It makes my blood boil. Those labels are alluring, but they are so deceptive. I often see products laden with toxic fragrances, sulfates, and other carcinogens in yoga studios, organic restaurants, and even the offices of holistic healers. Sadly, just because you are using a product that contains essential oils, it doesn't mean the product isn't formulated with toxic compounds and synthetic fragrances.

Air quality is not something you can take for granted, even inside your home and the personal spaces you inhabit. So what can you do to create healthier cleaning products for your home? First, make sure your rooms get ventilation. Second, if you like a natural scent, like basil, geranium, lemon, or pine, you can add these essential oils to your homemade cleaner—starting on page 87, I have supplied recipes you can tailor to your liking. But don't be surprised if your concoction doesn't smell exactly like the artificial basil and geranium you're familiar with in the synthetic-laden products you have been buying. You can also add essential oils to store-bought cleaning products, with a major caveat: the products must be truly all-natural, fragrance-free, and toxin-free.

Synthetic Scents

Sorry, but candles can also be a source of bad air in your home. That's because most candles are perfumed with synthetic scents. On top of that, the vapors that lit paraffin-based candles produce aren't meant for inhalation by humans—and it's easy to leave candles burning for hours, wafting soot, smoke, and other pollutants throughout your home.

If you love the convenience of scented candles and don't want to give up your wax habit, choose beeswax candles scented *only* with essential oils or natural fragrance instead. Just keep in mind that when you burn toxin-free candles, you are still burning off the essential oils they contain, so they won't have the healing benefits diffusing provides.

But the truth is, most scented candles, room deodorizers, air fresheners, and cleaning products are made exclusively with ingredients more harmful than we can imagine. According to the National Resources Defense Council (NRDC), most contain phthalates, those hazardous chemicals I mentioned when discussing the reed diffuser. While major fragrance houses are removing the phthalates from their scents, and companies like Johnson & Johnson are reformulating popular products to be safer and healthier for consumers, for now, it's better to replace these chemicals with natural alternatives, like essential oils.

The Effortlessness of Diffusing

Ready to start scenting your space all naturally? The easiest way to get started is by using a diffuser. Here are the basic steps before you begin diffusing:

THREE STEPS TO MAKING SCENTS FOR YOUR DIFFUSOR

1. *Purchase three low-cost oils in larger quantities.* Get the largest size you can afford (15 mL or larger) so you can use them freely. Again, be sure to buy organic or wild-crafted oils for your home. Oils like orange, pine, and fir are cost-effective, or buy extra of your primary oils. Look for oils stored in the European dropper bottles to make it easy to tap straight from the bottle. Here are two more of my favorite combinations using the primary oils:

To awaken: 6 drops lemon + 1 drop eucalyptus + 1 drop peppermint

To relax: 5 drops orange + 1 drop cedarwood + 2 drops lavender

2. *Select your favorite essential oil.* Find the one in your collection you absolutely adore or purchase a new one. This should be a scent that makes you feel good *every time* you smell it, so you can improve your mood instantly with the scent. A few suggestions follow. If you don't see your favorite on my list, get it anyway (see page 167 for what oils to avoid):

Awakening citrus: lime, grapefruit, lemon

Calming citrus: mandarin, orange, petitgrain bigrade, bergamot

Sensual flowers: lavender, geranium, clary sage

Grounding roots, resins: vetiver, vanilla*, frankincense*

Stimulating spices: basil, rosemary cineole, peppermint

Strengthening needles, leaves: spruce, pine, fir, hyssop decumbens* (do *not* use hyssop officinalis, since it contains neurotoxins and is unsafe)

3. *Choose two rooms to scent.* Decide which two rooms in your home you would like to focus on first and make sure you have the 100% essential oils or blends you need for those two rooms. (There are room-specific recommendations in the next section.) Please note that if you are doing a program, detailed in chapter 4, keep it simple: just choose from the list of oils recommended for the program you've decided to follow.

---

*These oils can be more expensive than others.

CREATE A WINNING COMBINATION

I always recommend making a blend of 100% essential oils as opposed to using them one at a time because of the synergistic effect of combining them. But using an individual oil to scent a room is fine, especially if you are using different oils in different areas of the house.

If you decide to combine two to three oils for your environmental scent, you will experience more benefits, however. When blending oils for your home or office, try not to be a perfectionist with your formulas. Instead, just let your nose lead the way. Smelling and testing out your blend is already a luxurious mind and body treatment in itself, so soak in the moment.

Here's how to make an easy environmental blend for the whole house: Choose two or three essential oils. Add more drops of the softer-smelling oil and fewer drops of the stronger-smelling oil. If you want a specific oil to stand out, adjust the number of drops to get what you want. One effective way to make your first time combining oils easy is to blend them in a glass first and then store the mixture in a dropper bottle or add to a selected cleaning product. As I mentioned earlier, always keep notes on your formula, so you can repeat it if you wish, and be sure to label the bottle with both the name of what you want to call the blend and the date you made it. It's really fun thinking up names!

It can also be helpful to set aside time to put together a unique combo on your day off (like a Sunday), adding one drop at a time until you have created a blend you really love!

If you're interested in buying a diffuser, there are two types I would recommend:

Sonic diffusers dilute the oils in water and use sound vibration instead of heat to diffuse. This is the type of diffuser I prefer because it can run safely for many hours, usually includes a timer, and it has an automatic shutoff when the water runs out. I use the Stadler Form jasmine aroma diffuser myself, since it's easy to clean and looks attractive. However, sonic diffusers all have plastic wells and don't work very well with citrus oils unless you clean out the diffuser with a cloth and a cotton swab between applications.

Nebulizers also diffuse oil without heat, like sonic diffusers, but they have a tendency to break. Nebulizers also are more difficult to clean, are more expensive, and tend to use much more oil. However, nebulizers are great when you want a strong medicinal effect.

Two other types I do not recommend:

Vaporizers use heat to create a flow of steam. The small ones can be worrisome because most brands are unstable and use high levels of electricity. Vaporizers have to be handled carefully, and heating an essential oil can change its chemistry and, as a result, the benefits you experience.

Clay pots, which heat with a tea candle, are a low-tech method, plastic-free, and typically sold anywhere you can buy essential oils. These have the same downsides as vaporizers because you are heating the oils. Also, the reservoir for the water and oil tends to become lined with a sticky film of reduced oils, which attracts dust, making these pots hard to clean, and eventually, you will start burning residue instead of your oil.

In general, I recommend avoiding diffusers that heat oils without water. Also, be wary of the oil included with a diffuser. Often these are low-grade essential oils or synthetic fragrance oils not suitable for your space. Every oil you use or inhale should be high-quality organic or wild-crafted.

TO DIFFUSE OR NOT TO DIFFUSE

A lot of people assume that you need a diffuser to add scent to a room, but that's definitely not the case. Essential oils, being extremely volatile, evaporate immediately. Their little microparticles become airborne as soon as you open the bottle. However, if your goal is to fill a large room or make a scent last longer, a diffuser can be a helpful tool. The basic guideline for all diffusers is not to diffuse essential oil for longer than one half hour at a time and wait one hour between diffusing sessions.

That being said, you should never diffuse the following essential oils: birch, black pepper, cinnamon bark, clove, ginger, lemongrass, oakmoss, and patchouli. Most of these oils are too strong, too spicy, or too hot, and they can irritate your skin and/or mucous membranes. Clove is among these potentially irritating oils, but because of its valuable antiseptic quality I will explain a safe way to use it to scent your home, provided you keep it away from young children.

Scenting Your Space, Room by Room

When infusing a room with beneficial essential oil vapors, there are other options to using a diffuser. You can add essential oils to toxin-free cleaning products or drop on nonabsorbent surfaces or natural (or organic) fibers. I hardly ever throw out an essential oil–soaked cloth or tissue since there is always a spot someplace in my home that needs refreshing. As you use essential oils every day, you will find that your home, your workspace, your body, and your clothes will automatically smell appealing and others will surely comment on it. I guarantee it!

When deciding which oil is appropriate for each room, go by what you like; although, as you'll see, I recommend stand-alone oils and oil blends I think work particularly well for every given room in your home. To test-run a combination, put a few drops of an oil on a tissue. Don't put drops of different oils on the same tissue; instead, use as many individual tissues as you need for each oil. Hold all the tissues near your nose to imagine a blend. Let your gut tell you what you want. Your preferences will change, but you can change which oil you use any time you need to refresh the air—so have fun!

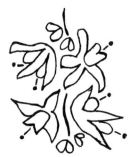

The Clean Bathroom

Key Oils

Peppermint

Eucalyptus

Cedarwood + spruce blend or fir (though less familiar than the traditional "clean" scent of pine, these needle oils will bring a whole new experience to "clean")

Clove (only 1 drop, and use it in a well-ventilated bathroom)

Tea tree and/or eucalyptus and/or thyme diluted in a cleaning product

Here's How

Wipe down the shower stall glass or bathtub surface with an unbleached paper towel dampened with your essential oil combo (4 to 6 drops).

Add 1 teaspoon of essential oils to your unscented, toxin-free bathroom cleaner, and use that mixture to clean your whole bathroom.

If you use vinegar-based cleaning products, follow with the essential oils cleanser to leave the fresh scent. Note:

If you use clove, only 1 drop is needed in your cleanser because this oil, which is a powerful germ killer, can have an overpowering scent.

Any time you take a bath or a shower and use your essential oils on your neck, shoulders, and chest, you are scenting your bathroom. Rosemary and peppermint in your conditioner will leave a lasting aroma, and they are supreme oils for hair care. Or you can tap 4 drops in the corners of the shower stall before stepping in, which creates the effect of an essential-oil-laced steam room.

Do not dilute essential oils in just water for cleaning! Even with their natural antimicrobial effect, eventually a water-and-essential-oils mixture will grow disturbing microorganisms that you don't want to spread around your bathroom. Either use 100% essential oils or dilute them in a cleaning product.

Why It Works

We tend to use strong-smelling cleaning solutions in our bathrooms to cover up odor. Clearly, hygiene is important, especially when ventilation is not always adequate. But these institutional smells mostly include chemicals not safe to inhale (just read the labels!). As natural germ killers, essential oils will keep your bathroom clean and refresh your senses. Since most have antifungal effects, they are perfectly suited for damp spaces. With all the bugs coming in and going out, using some of the most powerful, natural cleaning agents, like thyme and clove, will help your immune system stay strong. Instead of inhaling or applying these oils topically though, which can irritate the skin, reserve these oils for diluting in your safe cleaning products.

For the trio of antibacterial, antiviral, and antifungal features, eucalyptus, tea tree, and peppermint are stellar choices—all are strongly effective decongestants with many uses and are gentler than traditional cleaning products. Cedarwood is also noted for its antifungal action and spruce for its antiseptic, decongesting actions, including a hormone-balancing component. Together, these oils make great cleaning solutions and double as personal care oils you can add to a bath oil or salt scrub.

The Clean Kitchen

Key Oils

Lemon, lemon + lime blend

Grapefruit

Clove or thyme (only 1 drop)

Here's How

Add ½ teaspoon of a single 100% essential oil or oil blend to a sulfate-free, unscented all-purpose spray cleaning product and shake to mix it. Spray down your counters and sink after each meal. Let the spray sit on the surfaces for a few minutes before wiping it up.

For stubborn stains, pretreat the area with a few drops of 100% essential oils.

For cleaning natural wood surfaces, use cedarwood, lemon, or pine in your unscented product (do not use petrochemical-based wood products like mineral oil).

Why It Works

These upbeat essential oils help clear the lingering odors from cooking and are strongly antiseptic. Other oils that could work in your kitchen are spice oils, but I tend to think lemon is the great neutralizer, which is why I highly recommend it. Grapefruit is also a good choice if you tend to lose motivation in the kitchen, because it focuses the mind. And a combination of any of these citrus oils is especially cool and refreshing on hot days, when the kitchen can feel oppressive.

The Relaxing Living Room (or Den or Sunroom)

Key Oils

Petitgrain (clear) + clary sage (clear) blend

Lavender (clear) + coriander (clear)

Orange + Roman chamomile blend

Lavender (clear) + vetiver blend

Geranium + clary sage blend

Myrrh + frankincense blend

Tangerine + bergamot (clear) blend

Vanilla, benzoin, rose, rose absolute (must be organic; to save on cost, use only 1 drop of any of these to ease pent-up emotions after a frustrating day)

Here's How

Turn on your diffuser (to cover more space) already prepped with an essential oil or set the diffuser on a timer to turn on as you arrive home from work.

When you come in the door, grab a single 100% essential oil or oil blend of your choice, making sure it is a clear oil (see the oil choices listed), and tap a drop onto the wool or cotton fabrics in the room.

Tap a few drops of a single oil or oil blend onto any wool or cotton clothing you are wearing. Yes, even your natural-fabric clothes can act as a diffuser.

Why It Works

A main cause of both sleep and dietary issues is having trouble shifting gears when we get home. Often the time spent at work can be so intense and stimulating (or frustrating) that we can't calm down once we get home. We never shift into relaxation mode before our heads hit the pillow. When we have emotional stresses during the day, we may minimize or not have time to process. This disturbs both sleep and digestion.

In addition, being in work mode for long hours can become a rut we have trouble getting out of, even when our brains are tired. Simple tasks like preparing a dinner can feel too complex. And it can be difficult to be accessible and open to our families and/or loved ones when we have too much on our minds or unexpressed emotions.

Essential oils can help release and regulate your emotions (see the Relax and Focus program in chapter 4 for more information). Diffusing oils that soothe the nervous system helps you to release pent-up emotions and feel like yourself again. The oils I have listed for relaxing are primary for soothing anger, anxiety, and fear. Add an oil for digestive support, like coriander and/or mandarin. Bergamot is always helpful at the end of the day because it makes us happy. The sweet oils (vanilla, benzoin, and rose) are calming as well and especially helpful when you don't know why you are so irritable or quick to react. If you have trouble sleeping, be sure to do some reading or quiet activity in a room with these oils to prepare you for a fully restorative night.

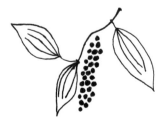

The Sensual, Sedating, or Awakening Bedroom

Key Oils

Sensual: coriander, jasmine, ylang-ylang, clary sage, vanilla, rose, sandalwood, patchouli + myrrh blend, basil + clove blend, and, to heat up the room, black pepper, cinnamon leaf, anise, ginger

Sedating: lavender + orange blend, anise + neroli blend, mandarin, clary sage, rose, valerian, spikenard + melissa blend (has a very strong effect), sandalwood, coriander, chamomile

Awakening: lemon + grapefruit blend, peppermint, eucalyptus + basil blend

Here's How

Sensual: Prepare your bedroom by tapping a few drops of a single 100% essential oil or oil blend onto a couple of decorative cotton or wool pillows before entering it. Never overpower the moment with an essential oil, and avoid scenting bedding and diffusing.

Sedating: Diffuse an oil or oil blend an hour before you go to sleep or right before you start your nighttime self-care rituals. Leave the diffuser on while you read, journal, or watch TV. When you're ready to turn off the lights, turn the diffuser off so the scent doesn't disturb your sleep. Also, if you need a sleep oil every night, have two favorite versions by your diffuser and switch between them every few days so you don't become desensitized to either.

Awakening: Diffuse the room upon rising to clear the air and inspire you. For a sunny waking-up experience, no matter what the weather, use citrus oils. To get more of a jolt, use eucalyptus or peppermint and add basil to round out the scent—these are dynamic brain sharpeners. If it takes you a long time to wake up, get all the help you can! Tap a liberal amount of a single oil or oil blend onto your cotton (or other natural fabric) robe in the morning and apply the oil topically or at the opening of your nostrils.

Why It Works

Sensual: Many essential oils are aphrodisiacs, so pick what you and your partner like. But remember: less is more. Essential oils that are too strong can be overwhelming or distracting and take you out of the moment. Be sure to keep these oils separate from your everyday oils (remember how associative oils are!), and alternate scents when an oil seems "stale" and you need something new. Feminine scents include clary sage, jasmine, and rose, but ylang-ylang and vanilla aren't for everyone. Sandalwood luxuriously relaxes and does well with warming spice oils, like basil, clove, or black pepper, to create a masculine combo that tends to heat things up!

Sedating: Essential oils are studied broadly for their sedating effect. You can count on getting results here. Just use them as directed. If one oil doesn't do it, try others and try the combos too.

Awakening: I have recommended oils that have a strong history of focusing the mind and putting you in a good mood. Again, use them with confidence and tailor them to your taste, and you will definitely feel the results.

The Fresh Closet (That Keeps Insects Away)

Key Oils

Geranium + lavender blend

Cedarwood

Peppermint

Lemon eucalyptus (eucalyptus citriodora)

Lime + peppermint blend

Here's How

Put as much oil as you like on a natural-fabric napkin, cloth, or wipe. It must be organic, or washed with a nontoxic detergent, so you don't pick up any harsh chemicals lingering in the fabric. Leave the fabric item on the floor of your closet and/or put it in your shoes (benefiting your feet as well).

Make your closet smell as strong or as subtle as you like, but make sure you like the scent enough to have other people smell it on you.

Put a cloth soaked with any of the key oils into your dirty laundry hamper and include the rag when you launder and dry the clothes.

Why It Works

Most essential oils are excellent insect repellents, especially cedarwood, peppermint, and lemon eucalyptus (eucalyptus citriodora). I discovered how much I loved geranium in the closet when I mistakenly spilled a bottle, used a rag to wipe it up, and just left the rag in my closet. When you add geranium to the classic scent of lavender, it creates a luxurious combo that makes your closet feel clean and soothing. But by all means, please consider your own favorite oil for your closet. Feel free to combine it with lavender, because pretty much everything goes with lavender. Your favorite in your closet takes the pressured feeling out of choosing what to wear. If you are not a morning person or you spend too much time making sure you like what you see and it makes you late, make your closet the first place to scent, so you start your day in a good mood. My wish is that you feel a wave of happiness come over you when you open your closet door!

The Healing Room (When You or a Family Member Has a Cold, the Flu, or a Cough)

Key Oils

Eucalyptus + niaouli blend (at the beginning of a flu)

Eucalyptus + ravensara blend (at an acute phase of a flu)

Lemon or grapefruit + hyssop decumbens (to keep the bug from spreading to your family)

Pine + hyssop decumbens blend (for allergies, fatigue, and to clean the air)

Cypress, bay laurel, eucalyptus (at the first sign of a cold)

Bay laurel (for a sore throat)

Spruce, fir, pine, cypress, benzoin (for a cough and to lift the spirits)

Here's How

Diffuse these oils in water.

Run the diffuser only as long as the sick person is comfortable with the oils, because we are more sensitive to odor when we are sick. Diffuse the oils in other parts of the home, away from the sick person, to reduce the spread of germs.

If you feel like you are coming down with a cold or the flu, to support your immune system's initial response, diffuse eucalyptus and niaouli (if you can't find niaouli, an aroma I prefer, use tea tree, which is easier to find but has a stronger scent).

If and when you become sick, switch to a eucalyptus + ravensara blend—this is a protocol chemist-aromatherapist Kurt Schnaubelt, Ph.D., recommends.

If you are already sick and you want to clean the air so others in your household don't get it, diffuse lemon or grapefruit with hyssop decumbens.

In preparation for and during allergy season, pair pine with a little hyssop decumbens to cleanse the lungs and strengthen your body's response to the deluge of airborne particles that trigger allergies. A drop of clove on a fabric swatch to place by your nose to inhale is a natural antihistamine as well.

Why It Works

It's hard to refresh air circulating in a room when someone is sick in their bed; you don't want cold drafts or perfumes around that person. But essential oils have you covered when it comes to cold and flu season, and using essential oils every day will boost your body's defenses. Diffused essential oils not only clean the air with their antimicrobial properties but can also speed up the recovery and healing process. In addition, essential oils have a mucolytic effect, which means they help your body clear out phlegm. For example, eucalyptus radiata clears out ear, nose, and throat congestion and is great for kids (five and up) too. Pine and hyssop decumbens clear the lungs and have an added benefit of supporting your adrenals, which, when depleted, create an equally depleted immune response.

Oils that help alleviate congestion are also great oils to use when you live in a damp or extremely humid climate. While conducting a spa training on the island of Nevis, I noticed that the high humidity caused every one of the therapists to experience chronic nasal congestion. You can imagine how much they loved my sinus blend, with eucalyptus, niaouli, and ravensara, when I gave it as a gift to all!

If you are sick, tired, run-down, congested, generally lacking in motivation, and/or simply feeling stuck in your life, mucolytic oils will lift you out of your funk and get you moving.

The Healthy and Productive Workspace

So many people talk to me about their mental fatigue, it sounds like the new epidemic. I keep repeating "To stay sharp, fuel the mind with oxygen, food, and movement!" But we have a hard time fitting in all three when our workdays are long and we need to stay productive—especially when we have to travel for work. When I was a dancer, two weeks before a performance started was when the whole show—the lights, costumes, music, props, steps, and promotion—all had to come together in an instant. During that time, I had to pick two out of the three things that made me perform well: food, sleep, and exercise. Luckily, as a dancer, oxygen and movement was a given. Trying to maintain healthy habits with a computer-centric lifestyle can definitely be a bigger challenge. (See the Relax and Focus and Travel programs in chapter 4 for more strategies to stay healthy and happy while at work or on the road.)

Key Oils

Lemon

Grapefruit

Lime

Bergamot

Peppermint

Basil

Cardamom

Rosemary cineole

Basil + bergamot blend

Lime + grapefruit blend

Lemon + peppermint blend

Rosemary cineole + basil blend

Here's How

Making a combo for your office environment is so easy—just blend oils in your blending glass, and you are good to go. You don't need a diffuser here because no one wants to overpower or annoy office mates.

Find a beautiful wineglass, brandy snifter, or large goblet you can keep on your desk. Keep three or four essential oils in a drawer in your desk. Upon arriving at work, place in the glass 2 to 4 drops each of whichever single oil or oil blend you want to use that day. Swirl the oils in the glass and hold the glass up to your nose. Practice slow breathing inhalations, with your belly relaxed to awaken your mind and put you in an inspired mood.

After lunch, add a drop of peppermint or a drop of cardamom (to focus) or coriander (to ease stress) to the glass for digestive support and so you don't get sleepy after your meal. Using these oils also creates the potential for more ingenious work! Inhale from the glass at the first sign of an afternoon slump, and refresh the blend if needed. Another inspiring oil is eucalyptus, especially if you tend to get allergies or congestion at work. As usual, choose what you love!

When you need to switch off from peppermint, use basil or rosemary cineole (be sure to check that you have the right type of rosemary). These are supergood brain fuel!

To shift out of work mode and prep for a relaxing dinner, tap a drop of anise, fennel, or coriander on a tissue with a drop of lavender and inhale this mixture ten times on your commute home, to stimulate digestion and let go of the stress of the day. Check for skin irritation on the crook of your elbow before applying any of these oils elsewhere topically.

If your office windows don't open, it's important to bring in as many plants as you can handle, such as a spider plant, Christmas cactus, or *Dracaena*. Once your plants are set up, bring in your essential oils. If the carpet in your office smells bad, purchase a cotton area rug and lay it over the carpeting from wall to wall. There are commercial desktop air purifiers you can try as well.

Why It Works

Essential oils help to purify the air, which can be especially important in commercial buildings and office spaces where off-gas is usually present. Off-gas is what results when toxins in a material—like wood, bedding, carpets, even children's toys—become volatile because the material in question has been treated with flame retardants, has a strong synthetic fragrance, or is made from composite building materials that use harmful chemicals to bond the different elements together.

Unfortunately, these toxins evaporate, cloud the air, and can be harmful to your health (like reed diffusers). Sometimes essential oils can interact with off-gases in the air and make the off-gases more toxic. When your environment is highly perfumed already and there is no fresh air, you are better off applying essential oils from the Breathing program (page 108) directly onto yourself: at the opening of your nostrils and onto your neck, shoulders, and temples to create your own shield of breathable scent.

Remember, your nose knows best. If you enter a space and it smells toxic, it probably is. If you feel like your space at home or work is taxing you more than it should, break out your oils, buy some plants, drink lots of water, eat as healthfully as possible, and open up as much ventilation as possible to freshen the flow of air. And make sure that you go outside for routine deep breathing breaks—refreshing for your mind, body, and definitely the spirit!

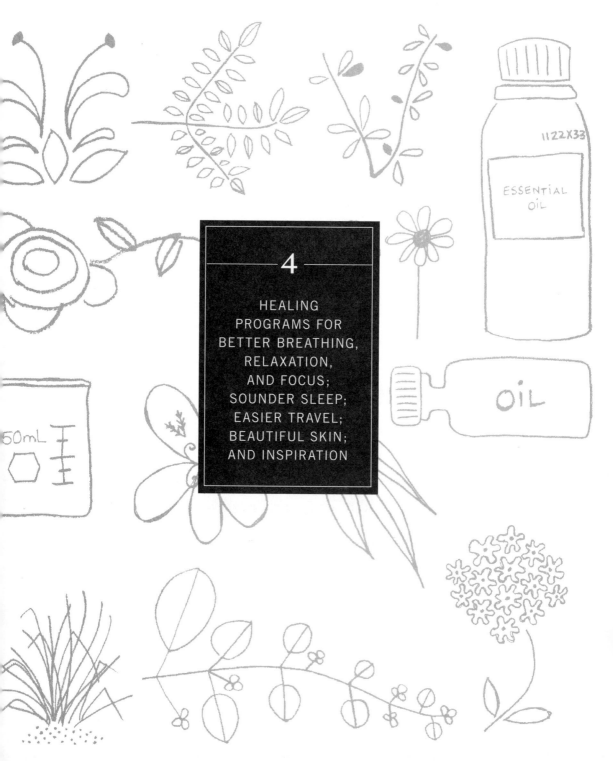

4

HEALING
PROGRAMS FOR
BETTER BREATHING,
RELAXATION,
AND FOCUS;
SOUNDER SLEEP;
EASIER TRAVEL;
BEAUTIFUL SKIN;
AND INSPIRATION

Now that you've learned how to make better choices about what to use in your environment, we can discuss how to remedy specific issues and ailments with custom programs. We often have an area of our lives that holds us back, causes us stress, or becomes a constant, recurring source of difficulty. When I first discovered essential oils, my back was that kind of problem for me. Even though I had come to New York to work as a choreographer, nothing could change until I found a way to remedy the pain and resume my life as a dancer. In our discussions about my health, I also explained my stubborn skin and digestive issues. Since these symptoms were triggered by the stress of my back pain, both the holistic massage therapist and trained aromatherapist I was working with knew that the back pain took precedence and we focused intently on finding a solution.

When it comes to using essential oils, being clear on what specific condition you want to focus on is crucial. If you attempt to solve everything that's wrong at once, you may select a combination of oils that don't interact well or simply make otherwise healing aromas another stressful part of your day. While it is great to dab lavender on a cut or inhale peppermint if you are nauseated, it is even better to have a central focus when using essential oils daily. By asking yourself "What do I need to focus on most?" and then selecting the appropriate remedy, you can see the immediate, remarkable benefits of incorporating essences into your daily routine.

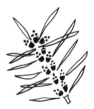

CHECK IN WITH PROFESSIONALS

In this chapter, I will help you pinpoint what issues you may want to focus on. However, this book cannot substitute for seeing a certified holistic therapist, acupuncturist, or aromatherapist. Find one in your area at the Alliance of International Aromatherapists: www.alliance -aromatherapists.org.

Please also bear in mind that all of the programs in this chapter simply offer lifestyle changes using essential oils as the catalysts. I am not a physician. I do not diagnose conditions, nor am I capable of prescribing specific solutions. If you are presently under the care of a holistic or allopathic health-care professional, especially if you are on medication, consult them before you start any use of essential oils. Their insights will be invaluable.

Similarly, it is always a good idea to check with your medical doctor before starting the use of essential oils, so you can safely rule out any unforeseen medical cause for your self-observations and experiences, especially serious conditions.

The reason we want to explore essential oils is the same reason we visit any health-care professional: to take care of our bodies and get on with the business of healing ourselves!

Using a program like the ones in this chapter will help you avoid ever feeling stuck or overwhelmed with too many choices. Instead, you will be prioritizing your needs and carrying out a plan to help remedy any negative aspects in your life. Even if all the programs offered in this chapter seem important or appealing, choosing one area to start focusing on will clarify your intention and help you feel better sooner.

This chapter offers six programs that show you how to incorporate the rituals in chapter 2 into a cohesive daily practice using just a few key oils. If you have already been exploring some of the daily rituals outlined earlier in the book, this next step will be an easy and natural progression forward. (And if not, now is your chance to get started!)

Please remember that you don't have to follow a program perfectly, do all the rituals that I recommend, or never miss a day. Far from it! By experimenting with the essential oils, you will learn what works and what's doable for you as an individual. (Not to mention that missing days can actually help your body learn how to adapt itself without the use of an essential oil, increasing the oil's efficacy the next time you do use it.)

The Programs—What They Are, How to Choose One, and How They Work

Start by reading each program description that follows. After reading, you may think something like *I need to do all of this?* No worries; you have plenty of time to try each one. But to begin, choose the one that sounds the most compelling, that you most *want* to do. You can always start with one program and shift to another at any point. There's also a Quick Start at the end of the chapter that you can begin right now with the oils you purchased after reading chapter 2.

Just like a gym workout, you will get better results if you change your routine on a semiregular basis. Typically, I recommend changing your program every time the seasons change. As the changes in weather and temperature trigger different responses in your body, switching essential oil programs can help you respond to those new and different needs.

The Breathing Program

If you have allergies, asthma, chronic sinus congestion, migraines, TMJ, tinnitus, or snore, or you simply get sick often, the Breathing program is for you. Additionally, if you frequently feel tired or stuck, or you have suffered a loss of a job, a friend, a family member, a pet, or your sense of purpose by putting others' needs ahead of your own, this program can be great. And if you don't know where to start, the Breathing program is a terrific, gentle introduction to using essential oils every day.

The Relax and Focus Program

This is the ideal program for busy people. If you frequently feel tense or stressed, injure easily, become irritable quickly, have anger issues, feel burned out, or can't focus, those are all signals that your state of mind may be holding you back. (This is also a great program if the Breathing program doesn't appeal to you.)

The Sleep Program

Living without adequate sleep is like not getting enough food, air, or water. If you have been getting less than six hours of sleep per night for two weeks, begin this program as soon as possible. It's best to nip a sleep problem in the bud to make sure you don't develop more serious issues. That being said, if your sleep problems are chronic, you may be too sleep deprived to get a good night's rest. In that case, it will be more effective to begin with the Breathing program or the Relax and Focus program before attempting the Sleep program.

The Travel Program

This program is specifically designed for people who travel often and find it challenging, for people who get anxious about travel way ahead of a trip, and for periods when you travel a lot (even if it doesn't seem to bother you that much). Also, if you sit for long periods of time without moving—which mimics travel—this can be a great program to use until you're able to introduce more activity into your routine. Prior to periods of travel, I recommend either the Sleep program or the Relax and Focus program so you're in the best shape to travel when the time comes.

The Skin Care Program

Essential oils are great "active ingredients" for superior results when it comes to any skin care product. For this program, I will show you how to make your own personal skin care products and cut back on the overload of products filling most of our medicine cabinets. If you are looking for a greener, more cost-effective way to get an ageless glow and still soothe your psyche, this is the program for you.

The Inspire Program

This program is for those who don't have a problem to solve per se. Maybe you just want to immerse yourself in the aromas of essential oils, explore something new, or rekindle your senses as you enjoy these beautiful oils. You may have a community of friends who want to do this with you. If you would like to explore new ideas and start planning a change in your life—a move, a home makeover, a new objective, a new job, a new approach to your health and wellness—this is a great way to start!

If at this point you haven't decided which program fits your current state, you can use my questionnaire to help you decide. (Or try the Quick Start at the end of the chapter.) If you simply don't feel ready to start a program, move ahead to chapter 5, where I'll show you how to create a small collection of oils for your medicine cabinet. Or just stick with your five basic oils from chapter 1 for now, trying out some techniques from chapters 2 and 3. There's no rush!

HOPE'S ESSENTIAL OIL QUESTIONNAIRE

Do you . . .

1. experience pain or excess tension in your neck or shoulders, lower back or hips, elbow or wrist?

2. feel numbness or tingling in your hands or arms, have difficulty grasping objects (like door handles), experience weakness in your hands, clench your jaw, or have TMJ?

3. feel overwhelmed or irritable, or have difficulty making decisions?

4. experience headaches, migraines, or mental or physical fatigue?

5. have sinus congestion, asthma, allergies, or sleep apnea, or snore while sleeping; or have you recently quit smoking?

6. experience insomnia, poor sleep, or anxiety that keeps you awake?

7. have tired legs, cold feet, or poor circulation?

8. feel thrown off when you travel, experience bad jet lag, or arrive home from a trip with a pulled muscle, a neck spasm, or insomnia?

9. feel like it's time for a change or need motivation?

10. feel burned out, stressed out, anxious, or depressed?

11. have sensitive skin, buy products that don't work for your skin, want to incorporate more natural skin care into your routine, or simply want to take better care of your skin?

The *Breathing* program is for you if you said yes to any question, but especially to 5.

The *Relax and Focus* program is for you if you said yes to 1, 2, 3, 4, or 10.

The *Sleep* program is for you if you said yes to 6.

The *Travel* program is for you if you said yes to 7 or 8.

The *Skin Care* program is for you if you said yes to 11.

The *Inspire* program is for you if you said yes to 9. (You can also start with the Breathing program if you are feeling low energy, and start the Inspire program once you get some of your pep back.)

Getting Set Up for Your Program

All the programs require a basic setup process first. Going through just the setup itself will help you feel focused, purposeful, and relaxed about your intention to use essential oils every day. Before beginning a program, you will need to:

1. *Purchase the key essential oils.* I've listed a few essential oils needed for each program. Buy those and a 4-ounce bottle of organic jojoba to mix your own blends.

2. *Read through the program and review the rituals.* These rituals are from chapter 2, so check earlier in the book if you need a refresher or have questions about them.

3. *Use single oils.* For each program, use a drop at a time. Or you can make an on-the-spot body oil by using a simple blending technique: place a few drops of the oil in your palm, add ½ teaspoon jojoba, and rub your hands together, then spread the mixture over the area recommended for your particular program. This also works well before you step into a bath, instead of pouring oil under the spigot.

4. *Make blends.* The full recipes for the oil blends in each program are in chapter 5. If you choose to use these recipes—and I hope you do—be sure to read through the ingredients before attempting to make a blend to ensure that you have all the oils on hand. I have selected a group of additional oils for each program to enhance your blends; feel free to read more about these oils in chapter 7. Blending is like cooking; the process is its own reward. I'm never as happy or as relaxed as when I'm making a new blend or following a recipe to re-create a blend I love.

5. *Design your personal scent.* You also have the option to formulate your own personal scent exactly to your liking (which I highly recommend!). For each program, I suggest some oils to experiment with while creating your personal blend as well. For more guidance on how to make your own formula, see the blending ritual in the Inspire program (page 135).

Note: If you are asthmatic or have allergies, test each oil separately before making your blend to make sure that the oil has the desired effect.

Start Your Program

Now that you have your rituals, blends, and individual oils to work with, start the program. As with all additions to your routine, it's best to choose a start date in order to set your intention and firm your resolve. The start date could be tomorrow, or maybe you want to start a program with a friend next week. However you want to adapt the program to suit your lifestyle is fine; just remember to use common sense and that, with oils, less is always more.

Each program contains these five options:

Start Your Day Out Right—a morning ritual, to set the day up right

Take a Mind/Body Break—an anytime ritual, to keep you on track

It's Never Too Late—an evening ritual to solidify your results as you rest and renew

Personal Scent—a ritual to set your intention and keep your focus

Help!—a ritual for when you need a quick fix or have completely lost track of your program or your sense of connection with your body

The goal of each program is to experience aromatic oils throughout your day, as a touchstone for self-care or self-healing. You may be thinking *How am I going to fit all these rituals into my life?* But take it slow, and do what you can in your own time. Give yourself rewards and praise for every step you accomplish. Once you get going with essential oils every day, the benefits you will feel will motivate you to create more time to continue exploring the program you've chosen. Start with just one ritual a day that's easy to incorporate. You can always try more techniques later. If along the way you realize that just one ritual isn't enough, that doesn't mean the ritual isn't working; it simply indicates that you should add another!

The Breathing Program

Key Oils *(Decongesting, Breath Relaxing, Energizing, Immune Supportive)*

Eucalyptus radiata or globulus (choose radiata for ear, nose, and throat issues)

Sandalwood or benzoin

Frankincense

Pine, spruce, or fir

From your collection: lavender, peppermint, and tea tree

The Setup

1. Purchase the key oils. Purchase these extras to enrich your formulations as your budget allows: orange, mandarin, cypress, rosemary cineole, myrrh, cardamom, petitgrain, and hyssop decumbens.

2. Use the key oils by themselves or make these blends:

Clear Your Head blend (eucalyptus, + rosemary + lemon; page 159)

ESSENTIAL OILS EVERY DAY   109

Clear Your Chest blend (pine or spruce or fir + hyssop decumbens; page 159)

Relax Your Breathing blend (sandalwood + petitgrain + lavender + mandarin; page 160)

Personal blend (make your own with frankincense, sandalwood or benzoin, and lavender, then add your choice from the extra oils in this program)

3. Review the rituals recommended in chapter 2.

Rituals

Start Your Day Out Right: Use the Clear Your Chest blend or a few drops of pine, spruce, or fir diluted in your palm during the Before You Step into the Shower ritual (page 58). Add the While Yawning ritual (page 58) to induce a nice long yawning sequence using a drop of lavender diluted in your palm.

Take a Mind/Body Break: Use the Relax Your Breathing blend or 1 drop of sandalwood in each palm. Push back from your desk, step away from

your work, or find a moment to be by yourself and practice the For a Quick Desk Break ritual (page 60). Later do the To Wake Up and Focus ritual (page 62), and then later the For a Tension Break ritual (page 63).

It's Never Too Late: First use the Clear Your Head blend or 2 drops of eucalyptus and do the Antisnoring Preparation ritual (page 69; even if you don't snore, this will clear your sinuses). After you have finished cleansing your face, use a few drops of the Relax Your Breathing blend with the After Your Cleansing Routine ritual (page 68).

Personal Scent: Use your blend or a drop of frankincense to anoint your collarbone, your clothing, or all your perfume points any time you want to smell your blend. Or use it during the For Daytime Meditation ritual (page 60).

Help!: Use the Clear Your Head blend or a drop of eucalyptus with the To Wake Up and Focus ritual (page 62) and clear your sinuses at the same time. Follow with slow breathing inhalations (page 52).

Why It Works

The oils in this program are designed to help you feel that you have more room to breathe. First, by decongesting—literally giving your lungs and sinuses more space—these oils clear out breathing passages and are also useful for soothing allergies, asthma, and sleep apnea. Second, these oils loosen the primary breathing muscles in your chest, ribs, and abdomen. (Of course, breathing begins in your nose and throat, and I have definitely geared the oils to this purpose as well.) They give you more energy while relaxing your muscles (such a perfect example of how essential oils adapt to your needs) and help move the focus of your energy from your head into your chest.

Here's a more thorough explanation of how this works: When we are under stress or in distress, we often have to concentrate for long periods. We may suddenly notice that we are transfixed by our thoughts (like a car racing around a track) or by the computer screen right in front of us. That's when breathing becomes shallow and tight. Expert Jessica Wolf calls this "screen apnea." "Of course, people at the computer are breathing," she told me, "but only the bare minimum. There's very little exchange of air. We breathe approximately eighteen thousand times a day, or an average of twelve times a minute. If we are only getting 70 percent of the oxygen on each breath, that's like losing five thousand inhales every day."

Breathing is paramount to life. We can go without food, water, or sleep for a time, but we can't stop breathing for more than a minute or two. Unlike eating or drinking, which require consciousness, we breathe whether we will it or not. Our breathing cycle is an ongoing process of oxygenating cells and expelling what we don't need. When we have proper oxygenation in our lungs, our minds are alert and our bodies have what they need to function. But without enough air, blood circulation slows and we lose energy fast. If you think the only or primary benefit of exercise is burning calories with a short-term release of endorphins, think again.

Exercise also keeps breathing muscles toned and flexible. Making the body and mind strong—there is no greater antidepressant than that!

The techniques in the Breathing program are designed to help you subtly retrain your breathing patterns to increase oxygen intake. Focusing on exhaling first, and relaxing the abdomen while doing so, creates deep, relaxed breathing. This is the best reset button for any stressful situation. Once you learn and practice this technique, it's possible to access the power of oxygen any time you want and to start feeling better right away. Over time, as you feel more grounded and energized, your voice will become more resonant, reflecting your state of renewed health. Not to mention that you'll experience a kick of confidence. There are so many benefits to breathing deeply.

THE BREATHING–POSTURE CONNECTION

A recent study shows the effect of good and bad posture. Whereas good posture increases serotonin, lowers cortisol, and instills confidence, poor posture does the reverse. Spending two hours a day with your head dropped forward toward your phone while you text or play games (instead of easily lifting your phone with your indefatigable biceps muscles!) is like carrying a twenty-pound kid on your shoulders for two hours every day. Clearly, this isn't something you would choose to do! However, that's not the worst effect of bad posture. Leaning over or slouching all the time also wreaks havoc on your cervical spine, giving you round shoulders and cutting down on your oxygen supply by 30 percent.

The Relax and Focus Program

Key Oils *(Calming, Focusing, Encouraging, Anti-inflammatory, Muscle Relaxing, Pain Relieving)*

Chamomile (German or Roman)

Basil

Geranium

Frankincense

From your collection: lavender and peppermint

The Setup

1. Purchase the key oils and include a few of your favorite citrus oils, the ones that make you happy, like bergamot, lemon, lime, or grapefruit. Choose bitter orange or mandarin if your digestion also reacts to stress.

2. If you intend to make blends, buy these extras as your budget allows: jasmine, cardamom, ylang-ylang, and vanilla absolute (this is not the cooking extract; see page 189 for more on absolutes).

3. Use the key oils by themselves or make these blends:

Focus with Calm blend (lavender + geranium + cardamom; page 160)

Strengthen Your Mind blend (basil + frankincense; page 160)

Relax Your Back blend (lavender + basil + chamomile + peppermint; page 160)

Personal blend (make your own with ylang-ylang, vanilla, or jasmine absolute + bergamot or other citrus oils you purchase)

4. Review the rituals recommended in chapter 2.

Rituals

Start Your Day Out Right: Do some yoga stretching in bed and then use the Focus with Calm blend for the Before You Step into the Shower ritual (page 58). To make your day even better, do the For Daytime Meditation ritual (page 60) with oils of your choice.

Take a Mind/Body Break: Use the Strengthen Your Mind blend or a couple of drops of peppermint, and push back from your desk to practice the For a

Quick Desk Break ritual (page 60). Later do the To Wake Up and Focus ritual (page 62), and then later the For a Tension Break ritual (page 63).

It's Never Too Late: Use the Relax Your Back blend or 4 drops of lavender diluted in your palm with the After Your Cleansing Routine ritual (page 68). Follow that with Relax Your Body Time (see sidebar page 115) and go straight to bed.

Personal Scent: Sprinkle your happy blend or a drop each of geranium and citrus oils on a tissue and inhale. Put drops on another tissue and toss it into your bag when you are going out. Put drops into your glass with the To Freshen Up Your Office ritual (page 60). Note: Instead of wearing this blend or oil, keep it to use as a mind refresher any time you need to change your mood, as often as desired.

Help!: Break out your peppermint essential oil and put a drop on the back of your neck if you can't think straight. Second option: Put a drop of geranium, vetiver, or vanilla in each palm—or combine two oils for a better effect—and do the slow

breathing inhalations technique (page 52) to soothe and release emotions.

Why It Works

The oils in this program are designed to help you bounce back from a period of extreme or prolonged stress. These oils have been linked to lowering cortisol levels by relaxing your body, slowing you down a bit, and revitalizing a tired or depressed mind. Though I am not a practitioner of Chinese medicine, I am inspired here by a TCM concept of blocked energy (qi) called "liver qi stagnation," which is used to describe a condition in which the liver has been stressed, not just by life's challenges but by our losing touch with our emotions as well. I see this all the time in my clients with pain. Many of us simply don't have enough time in the day to process all the emotional reactions that are part of normal life. These tensions can seem small (*Did he really mean to ignore me like that?*) but can easily build up. It's easy to get thrown off by someone slighting our work or being rude, or by a call from a sick friend or family member, but we often don't realize how negatively these moments affect us.

Once these small moments have built up to an untenable point, we find ourselves suddenly losing patience in a situation we would have easily handled before or feeling overwhelmed by the basic tasks of life. But worst of all, we lose our ability to prioritize and make the kind of smart decisions that help our days run smoothly—which can feel a bit like losing our optimism or a sense of positivity. When we live in this state over time, our body rhythms are upset: we don't digest food as well, we injure easily (both physically and emotionally), we crave stimulants and sweets, we become depressed, we lose sleep, and our muscles—especially in the neck and lower back—can lock up with tension. However, the oils I have chosen for the Relax and Focus program work together to help you break this pattern and return to a healthier state of mind (and body).

Essential oils flow straight up into the emotional part of the brain: your limbic system. At the end of the day you can use essential oils to release the pent-up emotions, so you can leave negative moments behind and sleep undisturbed.

Letting go becomes part of the natural rhythm of your days, and you no longer accumulate the emotional baggage that brings on anxiety or depression. Writing out your thoughts from the day, or talking them out, will help you go to bed with a clear emotional slate. Using essential oils to regulate your emotions can help you clarify what is important and, by calming your reactions, provide time to reflect.

When you inhale essential oils you are stimulating the autonomic nervous system to lower your blood pressure and slow your breathing while helping your mind to focus and self-regulate. I have chosen the essential oils in this program to help minimize mood swings and shift your body out of this constant state of feeling under duress. When combined with the rituals in this program, you can really make a change. If from this program you continue on with the meditation options in the Inspire program or spiritually grounding methods like yoga, tai chi, qigong, etc., all the better! Studies now indicate that you can even stimulate brain growth with daily routines like meditation.

RELAX YOUR BODY TIME

1. Before bed, apply the Relax Your Back blend to your lower back area.

2. Lie down, faceup, on a soft carpet, folded blanket, or exercise mat. If your back feels particularly tense, put a heating pad under your lower back.

3. Bend your legs so your feet are by your hips, hip-width apart—make sure your feet aren't sliding. If you feel you are tensing the muscles of your legs to keep them upright, you can lower one and then switch them after a few minutes.

4. Slide a one- to four-inch-thick soft paperback book under your head, not your neck. This will stretch your neck slightly. To relax your neck, let your chin drop toward your chest slightly. Try a thicker book at first. A light stretch is good, but if you feel too much stretch on your neck muscles, switch to thinner books until your neck feels comfortable.

5. Stretch your arms out to your sides, at shoulder height, on the floor. Bend your elbows and, keeping your elbows on the floor, place your hands on your lower ribs or abdomen.

6. Rest this way for five to fifteen minutes while visualizing your back heavily sinking into the floor—as if you were lying in sand and your back was making an imprint on the ground. At the end of the time, your spine will be stretched longer and your neck and shoulders will feel more relaxed.

7. Slowly roll over onto your side to sit back up, and get right into bed.

From a neurological point of view, the Relax and Focus program helps the body shift out of the fight-or-flight response into what Dr. Herbert Benson in the 1970s called the "relaxation response": the parasympathetic nervous system's recuperative state. This term is still used today to refer to the ability of the mind and body to calm through behavioral changes and mindfulness. We now know that stress isn't always a bad thing—it can be exhilarating, in fact—but the stress of our daily lives needs to be kept in check by triggering our relaxation response with some simple techniques and essential oils. So why not let essential oils help you keep your equilibrium?

The Sleep Program

Key Oils *(Sedating, Hormone Balancing, Very Calming, Anxiety Reducing, Fear Suppressing, Grounding)*

Clary sage

Spikenard

Mandarin

Petitgrain

From your collection: lavender and peppermint

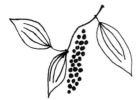

The Setup

1. Purchase the key oils. Add cypress if snoring wakes you up. Also, you can spice up your sleep blends if you substitute coriander and frankincense for clary sage and spikenard. If your budget allows, buy one of these luxurious, though costly, extras: rose otto, melissa, or neroli—all offer a welcome relief from a hard day. Buy them in the 2-milliliter bottle size—the luxury oils are worth it.

2. Use the key oils by themselves or make these blends:

Easy Day blend (petitgrain + clary sage + lavender; page 159)

Shift Gears blend (mandarin + clary sage; page 160)

Sleep Solid blend (spikenard + lavender; page 160)

Personal blend (make your own with the luxury oils and dilute it with jojoba)

3. Review the rituals recommended in chapter 2.

Rituals

Start Your Day Out Right: Use the Easy Day blend or dilute a drop of a luxury oil or frankincense in the After Your Shower ritual (page 59).

Take a Mind/Body Break: Use the Shift Gears blend, or any key oils you have on hand, in your glass in the To Freshen Up Your Office ritual (page 60). If you have a hard time slowing down at the end of the day, practice the When You Arrive Home ritual (page 67) and follow it with the tension-reducing Before Your Workout ritual (page 65).

It's Never Too Late: Use the Easy Day blend and do the Relax Your Body Time ritual (page 115) or a last stretch with the Before Your Workout ritual (page 65). After you have completely prepped yourself and your bedroom for sleep and you are in bed, use the Sleep Solid blend or drop any combo of your sleep oils on a tissue (except peppermint) and do the In Bed ritual (page 69). If you wake up, repeat the ritual. My rule of thumb: If you aren't asleep in ten minutes, use your oils!

Personal Scent: Take a moment to make your day dreamy and anoint your personal combination on your collarbone, your clothing, your hair, or all your perfume points, or do slow breathing inhalations (page 52) from your fingertips or a tissue, and/or do the For Daytime Meditation ritual (page 60). You can do this twice a day if needed. (Caution: Make sure these do not include the oils from this program's "It's Never Too Late" section; those must be used exclusively for bedtime.)

Help!: If you need extra help with sleep

(some minds are stubborn), put a few drops of peppermint on the tops of your shoulders at least one hour before bed. At first the oil will stimulate, but then the scent will leave you calm and relaxed.

Special Ritual: If snoring wakes you up, do the Antisnoring Preparation ritual (page 69) with cypress, keeping your eyes squeezed tightly shut and the water in the bowl at room temperature for this ritual.

Why It Works

Our parents worked long and hard to teach us one of our first life skills: how to put ourselves to sleep. But as adults, many of us need to relearn how to do it. The quickest way to regain this skill and reboot our habits is to use essential oils as part of our sleep rituals. Like Dorothy leaving Oz, we just need a little guidance (Glinda), an oil (the ruby slippers), and a meditative ritual ("There's no place like home"), and we can sleep like a baby again.

I have chosen oils that calm the psyche, soothe anxiety, and have a sedating effect when used at night.

When you use these oils during the day, you are actually helping yourself to sleep better at night. We have all experienced the way a vacation spot gives us access to better sleep. It's simple: when we are less keyed up during the day, we sleep better at night. Once you are sleeping better you won't need as much caffeine or sugar to sustain you through the day. That, in turn, will also help you sleep better. Eventually, you'll be able to simply do a nighttime ritual and be fine.

The grounding quality of these oils will slow your mind down, deepen your breath, and shift your focus to create beneficial sleep. This program includes rituals for better sleep and some practical guidelines that all the sleep specialists agree on. As always, use what works for you, but start first with breathing in the oils slowly.

After dealing with insomnia, it's often hard to believe that essential oils will work—especially when you have tried everything and nothing has worked. Even my mother was surprised when she had the best sleep with my blend. She was used to tossing and turning all night, but after inhaling my sleep blend, she woke up in the morning and realized there was just one beachlike imprint of her body in the sheets. She hadn't moved at all; she literally slept like a log. (See, Mom, my blends work!) The bottom line when it comes to the Sleep program is that the more time you spend awake in bed, focusing on your breath and inhaling the oils, the less time you will be anxiously waiting for sleep to come—and then it will.

THE BEST HABITS FOR THE BEST SLEEP

Address sleep issues sooner rather than later.

Since everything is more doable after a good night's sleep, look out for a pattern of sleeplessness. Letting sleep deprivation go longer than a few weeks could mean a harmful habit is brewing, which will ultimately affect your overall health, mental acuity, and safety. Essentially, if you have gone without quality sleep for more than two weeks, you are sleep deprived and should start this program to get back on track.

In addition, sleep specialist and neurologist Betsy Sherry, M.D., told me, there can be real physiological causes behind sleep problems, such as apnea, a deviated septum, and neurological sleep disorders. But the pattern of being an insomniac or being sleep deprived begins for most of us with hormonal changes, too much travel, a sick child at home, or anxiety and stress that goes unchecked until it becomes routine. Intervening with a few targeted lifestyle changes and a light-smelling, sedating blend of a few oils can be soothing.

A word to the seriously sleep deprived: Since you know your sleep problem is serious, I assume you know all the basics. But it doesn't hurt to repeat. Be responsible; anything less than six hours of sleep each night can impair your ability to assess risk and can put others at risk, especially when you are behind the wheel.

Plan your sleep like you plan your life.

• *Make your bedroom a sleeping mecca:* Block light with blackout curtains if you have to, remove buzzing electronics, charge your phone in the kitchen, and watch TV in another room. And definitely have your essential oils less than an arm's reach away. Set up an essential oil diffuser in your bedroom. Get it pumping to prep the room for sleep and then switch it off when your light goes off.

• *Less is more:* Switch to quiet mode an hour before bed, do the nighttime rituals in chapter 2, eat something small and drink a little shortly before bed so you don't wake hungry or having to go to the bathroom repeatedly. I have a client whose nighttime ritual takes one and a half hours and includes a long shower. Sometimes she complains about it, yet she has excellent sleep—talk about a gift horse!

• *Get into a rhythm:* Your body rhythms are controlled by light, so get in sync with the sun if you can. Try to go to sleep at the same time every night. If you routinely wake up every night for an hour, go to bed an hour earlier. While fitful sleep is not restful, nine elapsed hours with eight hours logged is a perfectly good way to sleep. And use a sleep mask to block light if you need to get more hours in the morning.

• *Get comfortable:* Select a mattress that is supportive and firm but not hard. If you sleep on your back, place one medium pillow under your head. If your back feels tense or sore, place a pillow or two under your knees. If you are sleeping on your side and you wake up with your arm asleep because you have been using it to support your head, this means you need to have more support for your head and neck. Most side sleepers need at least one pillow, if not two, to make sure the head is lifted off the shoulder. Instead of putting your shoulder on the pillow, gently lift your head and pull the pillow down to the top of your shoulder, then rest your cheek—not the back of your head—on it. If your shoulders feel tense or sore, hug an additional pillow. If your back feels tense or sore, put a pillow between your knees. Try not to sleep on your stomach. If you have chronic neck, shoulder, or lower back pain, these adjustments will help you protect sore areas from undue strain or compression while you sleep.

• *Cool down:* Our body temperature shifts at night. I worked with a kid who had a terrible problem because his body got so heated up at night. His scenario was feeling jolted awake, then sprinting out of bed to an open window and hanging his body out of it to cool off—he was pretty awake after that! So I gave him a blend meant to cool his body down (oils have temperatures—some, like ginger, heat your body up, while others, like peppermint, can cool you off), and I taught him how to relax his body before bed by breathing slower and deeper.

If you do get too warm at night, experiment with calming and sedating essential oils that cool you off during hormonal shifts or hot summer nights. Some examples of cooling oils that double as sleep aids include palmarosa, chamomile, and ylang-ylang.

• *Take the worry out of it:* What many people call insomnia stems from anxiety. I know that having too many worries before I go to sleep can lead to big problems at night, so I always try to prepare for sleep by putting aside my worries before I go into the bedroom. I might call my friends, watch TV, or read, but often a warm bath or meditation works better, because I'm resting my body, breathing slowly and fully, before attempting sleep.

• *Relax in bed:* Recent neuroscience shows that relaxing and even day-dreaming can be as restful as sleep. The key to feeling rested even if you can't sleep is to find a state of relaxation and calm—for your mind and body. Once you do this enough times, over the course of a week or a month or however long your body takes to learn a new habit, you will set up new neural pathways and no longer have an issue with sleep. One of the most common things I hear from clients who have used a sleep blend consistently is that, after time, it's unnecessary to complete the entire bedtime ritual, because just a whiff of their blend reminds their body to relax and their mind to quiet, and soon it's night-night!

• *Eat light:* Sleep is about resting and digesting. But you won't get the rest if you give yourself a whole new intake of ideas or foods right before you go to bed. As you are digesting your thoughts and feelings for the day, you are cleaning and cataloging. Your body is clearing out what you don't need (detoxifying) as you finish digesting the foods you have eaten throughout the day. So, basic rules for sleep: eat a few hours before bedtime and stay away from heavy foods that take longer to digest, like meat and heavy grains, as bedtime snacks.

• *Exercise during the day:* If you aren't active, that could be a missing ingredient to getting a better night's rest. If you are, be sure not to exercise too close to your bedtime, because it can disturb your sleep. I recommend a three-hour period before bed to slow down, shift gears, and gradually stop using electronics and doing any other stimulating activities.

Note: Essential oils don't block the restorative stages of sleep, such as REM, the way some medications do. However, if you are taking medications to sleep, don't stop taking them when you start this program. Instead, speak with your doctor about using the Sleep program to help wean you off these medications.

The Travel Program

Key Oils *(Diuretic, Mood Balancing, Hormone Adjusting, Liver Supportive)*

Litsea cubeba

Cedarwood

Grapefruit

Cypress

From your collection: lavender, peppermint, and tea tree

The Setup

1. Purchase the key oils. Optional additional regulating oils are clary sage, geranium, lemon, and grapefruit.

2. Use the key oils by themselves or make these blends:

Travel All blend (litsea cubeba + grape-fruit + cypress + cedarwood; page 160)

Time Out blend (cypress + lavender; or palmarosa + peppermint + lavender; page 160)

Personal blend (make your own using the optional oils in combination with other oils in this program, especially clary sage or geranium for the hormone-regulating benefit)

3. Review the rituals recommended in chapter 2.

Rituals

Start Your Day Out Right: Apply the Travel All blend or an all-over body oil of 2 drops each of litsea cubeba and cedarwood mixed (in your hand) with ½ teaspoon of jojoba. Follow this with the After Your Shower ritual (page 59) on the morning of your trip.

Take a Mind/Body Break: Use 3 to 5 drops of the Time Out blend on a tissue with ten slow deep inhalations for dozing once you are in transit. To soothe anxiety, use your personal scent with the For Daytime Meditation ritual (page 60). Bring an essential oil sanitizer, like a 100% blend of lavender and tea tree (in any proportions you like). These oils also double as a quickie air sanitizer and air filter for when someone beside you sneezes or jet exhaust fills the plane. To sanitize your seat, put a few drops on an organic cotton cloth and wipe down the seat, arms, buttons, and tray table. (This is so much better than a synthetic-fragranced wipe!) If you are flying on a plane, it's possible to get more blood circulation going by moving the heels of your feet up and down or simply sitting with your heels lifted so the backs of your legs aren't pressing into the seat. If you get an upset stomach, smooth 4 drops of peppermint on your abdomen in a circular motion on a bloated area (I always do this in the plane bathroom so as not to overwhelm my neighbor).

It's Never Too Late: Reapply the Travel All blend or your handmade body oil with the After Your Cleansing Routine ritual (page 68). Also, apply Travel All to your legs in upward strokes. Once you're in bed, if you still feel bloated from your flight, apply Travel All or a few drops of peppermint to your abdomen, smoothing the oil over the area (apply a thin coating of jojoba if you have sensitive skin), then follow that with a warm but not hot heating pad over your abdomen. To freshen up your hotel room, generously apply a single oil or oil blend to a cotton cloth and leave the cloth on your pillow. Sanitize your shower stall with a quick wipe of tea tree and lavender (antifungal).

Personal Scent: Anoint your personal combination on your collarbone, your clothing, or all your perfume points any time you want to smell your blend.

Help!: Use tea tree if you are worried about getting sick or if you need a quick jolt, using the daytime ritual To Wake Up and Focus (page 62).

Why It Works

Travel takes its toll no matter how much we strategize to minimize its effects. All of our body rhythms are influenced by light, climate, and our daily routine. Hormonal fluctuations, sleep, digestion, and energy levels are some of the rhythms upset by travel.

The oils in this section help your body adjust to the quick changes in temperature, climate, and time zone that are the main causes of jet lag. This program also includes some hormone-regulating oils to help your body rhythms get back in sync. Essential oils help speed up your physical adjustment to travel. This program also helps should you strain a muscle or end up with a tense neck from sitting in one position too long, because these oils are pain relieving, anti-inflammatory, and relaxing.

When we sit for a long time, blood circulation slows in our legs and we can experience swelling. For a small number of people who are at risk for deep vein thrombosis, this can be serious, but for most of us, this just makes us feel uncomfortable in transit and sluggish when we arrive. These travel oils are diuretic (a frequent solution for cellulite!), which helps decrease the fluid retention and indigestion that happens from sitting motionless for long periods of time. Sounds kind of like sitting at the computer without breaks, doesn't it? You can also do this program if you have been in meetings for days and need to get your blood moving but don't have time for a workout. The oils used in the Travel program are also emotionally calming on the flight and have all the immune-boosting properties you have come to expect from essentials.

If you travel frequently, never leave home without these oils!

TRAVEL MEDITATION PRACTICE

While seated in a desk chair, in a plane seat, on a train, or on a floor cushion, put a drop of a single oil or oil blend on each index fingertip. Close your eyes with an inward, downward gaze and simultaneously anoint your third eye and the crown of your head with the oil, pausing to imagine the place in your head where your fingertips would meet if they penetrated deeply. Inhale the remaining oil from your fingertips (or add more) with at least ten slow breathing inhalations (page 52). Relax the backs of your hands on your thighs and continue following your breath, repeating a mantra or silently counting each breath in your head. For a stronger effect, also anoint all along the bottom of your collarbone. If your mind wanders, you will eventually notice; without judgment, return to your breath. Layer the scent of the meditative oil when you travel by diffusing or by dispersing drops on a tissue within your on-the-move meditation space.

The Skin Care Program

My story of using essential oils for skin care is nothing short of miraculous. I had terribly sensitive skin growing up. As an adult, I sported either a rash, breakouts, or rosacea—my face was always a mess. Every conventional skin care product made my face break out, so I couldn't get facials. I tried to use makeup to conceal the eruptions, but that seemed to only make my face worse. I once tried every skin care product in a famous department store on Manhattan's Fifth Avenue, thinking that maybe I just needed more expensive products. But I had to return everything after a week, because they still didn't make a difference.

However, when I replaced all my products with essential oils mixed in a base of organic fatty oils, my problems went away in less than six months. Now when I tell people my story of how my face used to look, they are incredulous.

This program has a different format from the others, because most of us already have our daily skin care rituals in place. Instead of instilling new habits (like the other programs do), the Skin Care program focuses on switching out some of your existing products and techniques for refreshing new ones.

At first, changing out all of your skin care products may seem like a big investment. But remember, in the long-term you will save and benefit in a huge way. That being said, it is fine to do this program in stages so you don't have to purchase everything at once.

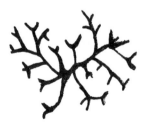

DON'T THROW AWAY YOUR BOTANICAL SKIN CARE PRODUCTS JUST YET!

But do throw away anything you purchased over a year ago and especially anything that contains preservatives, petrochemicals, and other harmful ingredients. Celebrity makeup artist, Burt's Bees spokesperson, and overall "green" cosmetics expert Katey Denno put together a perfect list of no-nos for her green makeup workshops and clients, like Amber Heard, Amanda Seyfried, and Alanis Morissette. (See page 224 for the full list of no-nos). This is a great guide to follow when reimagining your skin care products and routine. If you see any of these chemicals listed as ingredients in the products you are currently using every day, those are the ones you need to phase out first. The health risks from repeated, long-term use of these products is not worth it, especially if you are already seeing skin problems you can't resolve.

Selecting your oils is important. You will need to choose your key oils according to your skin type. However, if you are unsure which oils to choose, don't worry; I have selected oils that, regardless of skin type, will work for everyone. I recommend you experiment with different oils to see what works best for your individual skin. If you have acne or an oily skin type, you may need to pay more attention and experiment. If you go regularly to a dermatologist or aesthetician, ask them for their recommendations. (I also do not address more specific skin conditions, like eczema or dermatitis.)

Once you switch to more natural skin care rituals, the problems you face now may simply resolve themselves. As we learned in chapter 1, a variety of rich emollient fatty oils, such as argan, rosehip seed, or even olive oil, can be combined with essential oils to create natural skin care products, but jojoba is best for both face and body. It doesn't clog pores and it closely matches the oil your body produces (called sebum). It's appropriate for any skin type, including acne-prone skin.

Jojoba oil is made from the seeds of a robust desert evergreen shrub, the jojoba plant. Because this oil has a longer shelf life than other fatty oils, I recommend always keeping an ample supply of it on hand. It is the premiere oil for natural hair care. I'm so pleased to share that you don't have to spend extra money purchasing products like the synthetically loaded, artificially scented Moroccanoil products that I see in hair salons everywhere. Instead, it's easy to make a superior hair care product yourself. Add some sandalwood essential oil to your jojoba oil and voilà! This combination can be used as a styling tool or as an excellent scalp treatment that creates healthy, shiny hair.

Jojoba is also the best to use in your essential oil personal scent, because unlike perfume (which is usually made with alcohol, which disperses the scent and isn't beneficial when inhaled), jojoba mixed with essential oils creates a personal, breathable, intimate scent that attracts with more subtlety. I always love the moment when I hug a friend and they say, "Oh, you smell so good!" And it happens a lot.

Key Oils

Buy organic oils whenever possible. It's the only way to know for sure that you aren't putting pesticides in your skin care products by accident.

For Acne-Prone and Oily Skin

Face oil: lavender, ylang-ylang, and/or petitgrain

Hydrosol: lavender

Cleanser: lemon or grapefruit

Scrub and/or mask: clary sage, carrot, and/or vetiver

Spot treatment: tea tree

For Sensitive Skin

Face oil: neroli, German chamomile, and/or palmarosa

Hydrosol: neroli

Cleanser: geranium + carrot

Scrub and/or mask: ylang-ylang

For Pallid, Lifeless Skin

Face oil: rose otto, jasmine, and/or ylang-ylang

Hydrosol: rose

Cleanser: grapefruit

Scrub and/or mask: rosemary verbenone

For Dry and/or Mature Skin

Face oil: geranium, sandalwood, and/or clary sage

Hydrosol: neroli, rose, geranium, or sandalwood—your choice

Cleanser: palmarosa

Scrub and/or mask: Instead of an essential oil, use an emollient blend of olive oil, avocado oil, and manuka honey (antibacterial and humectant).

For Healing Skin (Scabs, Wounds, Sunburn, or Inflamed Skin)

Face oil: helichrysum, carrot, German chamomile, and/or frankincense

Hydrosol: helichrysum

Cleanser: unrefined coconut oil + neem oil with lemon, lavender, and myrrh

Scrub and/or mask: Avoid until healed, except when using pure aloe vera to soothe a sunburn

Face Oil Base

For *sensitive* or *pallid, lifeless* skin, use 1 tablespoon olive oil, 1 tablespoon jojoba oil, and ½ teaspoon rosehip seed oil, which is regenerating.

For *acne-prone* or *oily* skin, blend 1 tablespoon jojoba oil, 1 tablespoon grape seed oil, and ½ teaspoon evening primrose oil, which is hormone balancing and anti-inflammatory.

For *dry* and/or *mature* skin, use 1 tablespoon olive oil, 1 tablespoon avocado oil, ½ teaspoon rosehip seed oil, and ½ teaspoon argan oil, which prevents moisture loss.

For each face oil base, add 12 drops of your key essential oils. If you make your face oil in large batches, store the bulk of it in the refrigerator.

For all skin types, you can also add to your face oil a topical antioxidant, antiaging booster: ½ teaspoon pomegranate oil or a few drops of mixed tocopherols (vitamin E) during periods of stress.

If your skin is affected by changing climates or seasons, or by travel, adjust your face oil base as follows:

During *hot weather*, substitute 2 teaspoons of the olive or jojoba with grape seed or kukui oil.

During *cold weather*, substitute 2 teaspoons of the jojoba with argan, avocado, or coconut oil.

Cleanser Base

For *dry, mature,* or *sensitive* skin, use olive oil.

For *acne-prone* or *oily* skin, use a charcoal soap or a botanical cleansing gel (see the resources section), preferably unscented and not drying, which would stimulate more oil production (test first without adding an essential oil).

For *pallid, lifeless* skin, first use olive oil, removing dirt and makeup with a soft cloth, and then use a botanical cleansing gel. Apply both with upward, circular strokes, which works like a quick version of the Face Massage ritual (page 133).

For each cleanser base, put ½ teaspoon in your palm and add 1 or 2 drops of your key essential oils.

Scrub and/or Mask

For *scrubs,* start with a face oil application, then mix 1 teaspoon scrubbing granules (preferably colloidal oatmeal—see the resources section—and never the banned microbead product) with enough water to make a soft paste and apply in a gentle, upward circular motion, avoiding eye area.

For *masks,* start with a face oil application, then mix 1 teaspoon powdered clay: white, green, or pink with enough water to make a soft paste and apply. Remove with a soft damp cloth before the mask dries.

Optional: To moisten scrubs and masks, add manuka honey for its healing and moisturizing properties.

The Setup

1. It's an investment up front, but for long-term savings, purchase the essential oils and the hydrosol that match your skin type and the ingredients for the face oil base, cleanser base, scrub, and mask and store them in your refrigerator.

2. Since each batch of your face oil should last no more than four months, you can change it as the seasons change—another bonus of using essential oils that ready-made skin care lines can't match!

Rituals

Start Your Day Out Right: Follow a morning pre-makeup ritual.

• Spray your face with a hydrosol. (If your skin is oily, you can use your cleanser first, but keep in mind that too much washing will only stimulate more oil production. Try it both ways.)

• While your face is still damp, apply a face oil blend. Put 3 to 8 drops on your clean fingertips, rub them together, and press them around your eye area, then lightly sweep your fingers up and out on your face. Do the Face Massage ritual (page 133) to reduce puffiness, increase skin tone, and start your day relaxed.

• Spot-treat blemishes with tea tree or lavender.

• Now you will need less makeup since your skin will be glowing!

Take a Mind/Body Break: Using your choice of hydrosol, spray your face anywhere, at any time. Hold the sprayer four inches from your face when spraying. Blot the skin with a tissue and reapply face oil around your eyes, tapping lightly using your ring fingers on the bones around the eye, not the eye area itself.

It's Never Too Late: Follow a nighttime cleansing ritual.

• Combine ½ teaspoon cleanser base and 1 drop of essential oil in a clean hand, rub your hands together, and smooth your hands over your face, moving your fingertips up and out and circling your eyes, taking care not to get oil on the lashes. Wipe off excess oil with a wet organic cotton wipe (washable). Substitute a botanical cleansing gel if your skin is oily or has acne. If you have broken skin, use warm water to gently remove the cleanser, never rub your skin with a washcloth, and spot-treat with essential oils. Do not dry out oily or acne-prone skin with excessive washing; as I mentioned before, this will only stimulate the pores to produce more oil.

• Mix scrubbing granules with your hydrosol and press the mixture onto your face. Gently remove the granules with warm water and a damp wipe.

• Spritz your face once more with the hydrosol and blot it.

• Apply your face oil blend. If you didn't have time for a facial massage in the morning, do it now.

Help!: Apply a mini facial (choose a steam and/or a mask).

• *Steam:* Pour heated, but not boiling, filtered water into a bowl. Add 2 drops of lavender to the water and lean your face over the bowl. Let the steam deeply clean and soften your skin so the dead skin sheds without scrubbing. Follow this with a spray of hydrosol to tighten the skin and then apply your face oil. The face oil protects and moistens your skin before the mask if you have time to do both.

• *Mask:* After cleaning your face, mix filtered water with powdered clay into a loose paste. Add some manuka honey if desired, especially if your skin is dry. Pat the mixture on your face and neck, avoiding the eye area, and lie down until you start to feel the mask tighten but not dry completely. Remove the mask with damp, cool cotton wipes. Follow this with a spray of hydrosol to rebalance the skin and remove any extra mask material, and then apply your face oil (a second time if you did the steam).

• Follow these treatments with your choice of an organic lip balm, and spot-treat any inflamed areas or blemishes with a drop of 100% tea tree or lavender applied to a cotton swab. Wait for at least an hour before applying makeup.

Why It Works

If you are looking for a purely botanical antiaging program for your daily skin care, look no further than essential oils. Essential oils not only deliver much needed antioxidants that our skin requires to handle environmental stressors but also support new cell growth to regenerate the skin, encourage healthy collagen, and cleanse lymphatic fluid buildup in the facial and neck tissues (see sidebar), which makes skin look puffy or lifeless. Given you are hydrating adequately by drinking water, essential oils penetrate deep below the skin's surface to nurture the very foundation of radiant beauty. Using essential oils will not only keep your skin supple and tight but also help to heal wounds faster and with less scarring.

Traditional creams and lotions sit on the surface of the skin. They work by pulling moisture from the air to the surface of the skin, which causes a short-lived appearance of smoothness that wears off as the day progresses. These products typically have only one or two "active" ingredients in a base of inactive ones (and why would we want that?). Essential oil skin care *only* contains active ingredients. Mixed in a base of organic vegetable fatty oils, this type of skin care also provides the vitamins A, C, D, and E, essential fatty acids, and other nutrients our skin needs—naturally. Since botanicals work with our hormones, essential oils can easily be tailored and changed as you age and as the seasons change, and they can even come to the rescue during a period of swings in your bodily rhythms or life in general, like when you travel or go through extreme stress.

Often we wear stress on our faces. Why not use essential oils to reduce the stress we feel and slow the signs of aging while boosting natural beauty?

FACE MASSAGE RITUAL

This massage helps move lymphatic fluid, which can become trapped in tissues due to stress, and it is adapted from the Joanna Vargas Skin Care blog. Practice this slowly and mindfully, perhaps while sitting down instead of standing in front of your mirror. This ritual increases awareness and teaches you how to be gentle when touching your skin:

1. After applying your face oil to your face and neck, put your fingertips together and place them just above your collarbone. Move them in slow, smooth circles along the top of your collarbone for one minute. This technique of slow, circular fingertip massage continues throughout. If you have spots that feel inflamed or sensitive, be extra gentle and don't press on them with your fingertips.

2. Move the massaging slowly and incrementally up your neck and throat area to your ears.

3. Massage under your chin, pushing the fluids along the underside of your jawline toward your lymph nodes on both sides of the front of your neck and then behind the ears to the lymph nodes at the base of your skull. Again, be careful not to irritate sensitive areas.

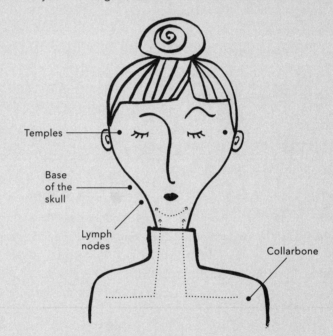

Temples

Base
of the
skull

Lymph
nodes

Collarbone

4. Continue this massage technique on your face, going from front to back and then pulling the fluids down to your jawline.

5. Repeat step 4 and then finish with your fingertips on your temples for a slow, circular mesmerizing massage. You may notice your eyes will be watery, which is good! The eye area will be less puffy as well.

The Inspire Program

Key Oils

• *Base/lower body notes* for concentration (which slowly evaporate over the course of a day). Family theme*: frankincense, sandalwood, patchouli. Health theme: spikenard, vetiver. Love theme: cedarwood, rose with ylang-ylang. Romantic love theme: jasmine. Career theme: geranium. Wisdom theme: myrrh.

• *Middle/heart notes* for meditation (which evaporate over six hours).

---

*The matching of specific essential oils to concerns that become our lifelong themes is a type of treatment called constitutional therapy in Traditional Chinese Medicine. I was introduced to this approach by my teacher, himself a Taoist monk. He called these lifelong constructs "palaces," similar to the Bagua map used in feng shui. He explained that healing with essential oils matched to these palaces is not physical, science-based medicine, but vibrational medicine based on plant essences that embody the vibrational energy of the plants. By focusing on a theme to resolve the recurring issue instead of seeing each concern as an isolated problem to push off, we can move on with a greater sense of freedom and happiness. Daily ritual with essential oils offers that focus. I have used these themes to guide my clients, and myself, as I have moved into different phases of my life. They bring more perspective and inspiration to the process, and I can only tell you that wonderful changes have followed. Doesn't this remind you of the early days of essential oils and incense . . . through smoke we gain clarity?

Prosperity theme: coriander. Career theme: benzoin, melissa. Wealth theme: helichrysum and/or rosemary.

• *Top/head notes* for elevating the spirit (which evaporate quickly, within three hours). Travel theme: fir, lavender, basil, bergamot (don't wear this outside in the sun, because it's photosensitizing), tangerine or mandarin, and/or orange.

The Setup

1. For this program, pick three to five key oils that are compelling to you, including at least one from each note. Purchase your oils in 5-milliliter dropper bottles. Instead of following a formula, make your own blend by picking one from each group, or note, listed in the key oils section, and add these oils to a base of jojoba. Ultimately, you can make your blend as strong or as diluted as you want, to fit your desire and to please those closest to you (it's a good idea to ask if your blend is too strong or too weak, or even simply if it smells good to your friends, partner, and family!). Use your senses and your intuition to choose which oils intrigue you. If

you aren't able to smell the oils in person, order samples of what you are considering (Eden Botanicals has an excellent sampling system). Smell the oils, read about them in chapter 7, and allow some time for what you've read and smelled to merge. Here are a few suggestions to help you with the selection process:

• Include an oil that corresponds to your life theme or palace.

• If you want to let go of attachments, use more of the top note oil.

• If you want to concentrate better, use sandalwood.

• If you want to feel protected and more open to possibilities, use myrrh and geranium.

• If you want to give more time for truths to be revealed, include vetiver. You can experience this effect even before you have put together the whole blend; just put 1 drop in the crook of each elbow. Smell the vetiver the next day, before showering, and without reapplying it; notice how the aroma has changed and how your psyche responds to it.

Instead of following a formula, make your own blend in a blending ritual. To start, I recommend clearing out quiet space and time for the blending phase, if at all possible.

Blending Ritual

• Put a drop of each chosen key oil on a separate tissue. Hold all the tissues up to your nose at the same time to smell the blend. If the smell of any particular oil is too strong, hold it

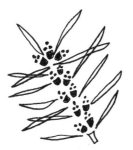

farther away—this will be the oil that you want to include less of. Decide on a middle note to be your primary oil—the one you want the blend to smell like.

• Write down a rough approximation of what you include as you blend it. You will start with the middle note, roughly adding these quantities I suggest.

• 20 to 30 drops of your primary, middle note: This is what your blend will smell like. Place the drops in a glass, swirl, and inhale to get a full sense of the aroma.

• 5 to 15 drops of your base-note oil: First add 5 drops to your glass, then add 1 more drop at a time until you have the right amount. Swirl and inhale to get a full sense of the aroma.

• 10 to 20 drops of your top-note oil: Similar to your base-note oil, start with adding 5 drops to your glass, and add 2 more drops at a time until you have the right amount.

• Add more of the primary oil to your blend until you have exactly what you want and then transfer to a 10-milliliter roller bottle.

• Leave the blend for a day and then return to it for final adjustments, filling the bottle with jojoba and tilting up and down to finish blending.

• When it is done, label and keep it with you on your desk, in your purse, or in your backpack. Use the roller to anoint the blend on your temples and other points near your face.

Rituals

Reminding Your Mind: Use this oil blend as a trigger to return to your intention throughout your day. Your focus will help you steer your choices and alert you to new opportunities. Here's how: Anoint your body at least once a day and up to five times, depending on how strong the aroma is and how often you need reminding. Some options for where and when to apply it include in the morning with the After Your Shower ritual (page 59), in the evening with the To Switch Gears ritual (page 68), or during the For Daytime Meditation ritual (page 60). Or simply anoint your personal blend on your choice of your collarbone, in your hair, on all your perfume points, in the crooks of your elbows, between the eyebrows around your third eye, in the center of your chest on your sternum, or on the crown of your head. Each time you use it, let the oil remind you of your intention.

Seated Meditation: To use your blend with a meditation practice, explore a meditation tape, a course, or an app, or go to a meditation center. Seated meditation is optimal, but there are many kinds of mindful activities, from swimming, where the sound of the water and the bubbles from your breath becomes hypnotic, to arts and crafts like watercolors, knitting, or ceramics, where the calm focus on process and the rhythmic movement of the hands

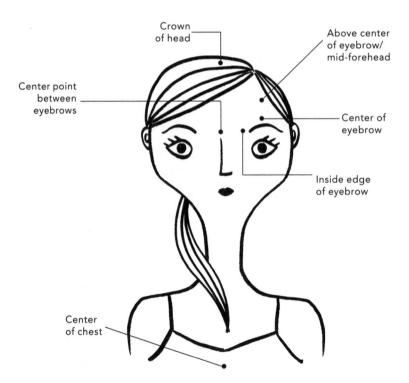

Crown of head

Above center of eyebrow/ mid-forehead

Center point between eyebrows

Center of eyebrow

Inside edge of eyebrow

Center of chest

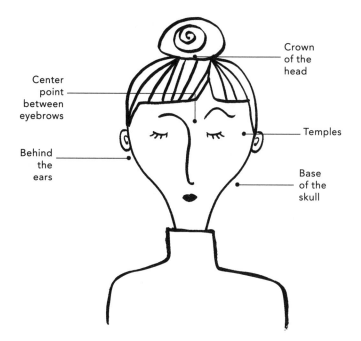

Crown
of the
head

Center
point
between
eyebrows

Temples

Behind
the
ears

Base
of the
skull

relaxes the psyche. Begin with slow breathing inhalations (page 52) of your Inspire program blend and the For Daytime Meditation ritual (page 60). An essential oil can work like an affirmation, clearing your mind of distracting emotions to make it easier to meditate.

Adagio—A Grounding: Solvitur ambulando ("It is solved by walking"). Being in nature is our refuge, a place where we can experience quiet and peace, and get out of our heads, where the light, odor, and feel of where we walk grounds us. Walking silently in nature helps us notice that the world inside our heads might be a very tight spot. For this ritual, anoint your Inspire program blend on your temples, the crown of your head, behind your ears, and at the base of your skull. To allow for a shift and a sense of fulfillment, let the oils calm your spinning thoughts and deepen your breath.

A camping trip, a walk in the mountains, a hike up a trail, or a swim in a river or lake (especially swimming on your back looking up at the sky) can make one hour feel like a complete vacation from the buzz in your brain. As you feel the movement under the soles of your feet, and your breath sustaining every step, your senses will reawaken and you can finally expand your thinking.

Why It Works

We spend too much time looking forward, focusing on our computers, only walking with purpose, using our hands right in front of us, for our imaginations to be sustained. When we feel a need for change, feel stuck or burdened by responsibility, we need a way to expand our perspective. Using essential oils to expand the senses while being outside in a natural environment is a very useful (and proven!) therapy. I encourage you to explore the oils you love, creating your own breathable perfume and taking it on a trip somewhere, even if it's for just an hour. Making this ritual a touchstone for your vision and an intention of what you want to come next can help you stay in touch with yourself and your body.

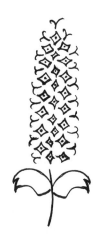

The Quick Start Using Only Primary Oils

You can do a quick start in lieu of a full program with just your lavender, peppermint, lemon, tea tree, and cedarwood oils or with the substitutes geranium, grapefruit, eucalyptus, and frankincense.

1. Explore a morning ritual using your tea tree oil to promote alertness.

2. Explore a daytime ritual using your peppermint oil to focus, relax, breathe more deeply, digest more effectively, and relieve pain.

3. Explore a nighttime ritual from "At Night: Essential Oils to Shift Gears, Slow Down, and Sleep" (page 67), using your lavender oil to care for your skin, soothe anxiety, and promote sleep.

4. Do the For Daytime Meditation ritual (page 60) when you exercise or do yoga; this is a great place to add in a little extra self-care.

5. Pick a program and buy just a few of the key oils first, to confirm you have chosen the right program.

6. Gradually acquire the extra oils.

7. Start using blends following formulas instead of using one essential oil at a time.

8. Finally, indulge and make your personal scent(s).

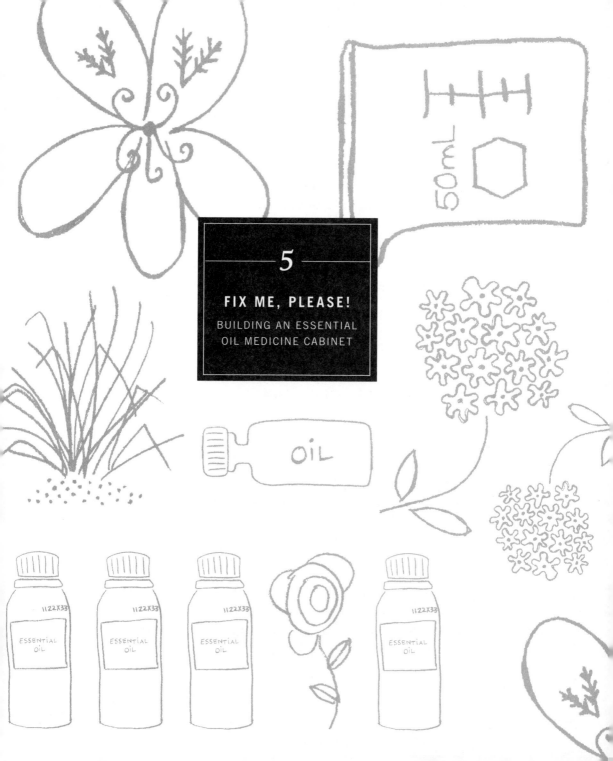

5

FIX ME, PLEASE!

BUILDING AN ESSENTIAL
OIL MEDICINE CABINET

My dearest friends jokingly call me Dr. Hope. But in truth, I love teaching people how to take better care of themselves. Nothing gives me more pleasure than hearing how someone cured a malady or made a lifestyle change for the better. I want to know all the details.

When I started dancing at the age of six, I became obsessed with self-maintenance. My training prepped me for a lifetime of strong muscles and physical self-awareness, but none of us is immune to the influences of our family's history. My beloved family is a relatively homogenous group of high-strung workaholics and perfectionists. We're very intense people who keep going like Eveready batteries until we end up with a health problem. I wasn't spared these tendencies, but as a dancer, getting sick was out of the question. Over the years, as I found myself following my family's lead, passionately adding more and more projects to my agenda, it often felt like I had "the curse of the Gillermans." When it comes to my health, I have had to constantly challenge myself to remember what I knew about stress and intentionally seek new ways to disrupt those ingrained Gillerman habits. And for this I am grateful. So my studies continue.

One thing I have learned over and over from my clients and my own trials is that extreme effort, extreme exercise, extreme diets, extreme self-denial, extreme discipline—really, extreme anything—always comes with a price. And yet, just like so many of us, I still tend to overdo it, despite seeing obvious warning signs, such as breathing shallowly, making mistakes, or having a minor accident, like stubbing my toe. Today, when I find myself with too much on my plate—or start to show signs of constant stress and anxiety on my face—friends and family members remind me, "Hope, you know what to do!" That's when I check in and tell myself, "You can't sacrifice your health; just breathe, get grounded, and do what you know best." When I was younger, I used to "cure" myself with dancing. As an adult, I go to my oils.

Over the years, essential oils have helped me overcome my predisposition toward rashes, eczema, rosacea, lower back pain, IBS, thyroid issues, weak lung qi, and a baseline of anxiety matched with depression. Some of these health challenges were major obstacles for me, and some I sidestepped completely. But each time I met a health issue with a thorough, holistic approach, the issue was resolved. Using essential oils has cleared my skin, aided my digestion, increased my energy, boosted my immune system, and supported my mental health. I have never been an insomniac, but I always keep essential oils by my bed, for whenever a sleep issue arises. When injuries from dancing, yoga, scoliosis, or foolishness crop up, I am able to resolve the pain without surgery or meds. I simply create a healing blend and pay attention to my body's signals. I intend to live the rest of my life pain-free (or at least without chronic pain).

Every time a problem—mental, emotional, or physical—crops up, I do two things: First, I ask myself, "What is really bothering me?" Am I feeling pain, bothered by anxiety, not sleeping? As I ask these questions, I talk to the go-to people in my life, to get a better perspective. When Mom suggests something as tried and true as "Take two aspirins and go to bed," I do a simultaneous translation for how that would work with essential oils and reach for my blend that is muscle relaxing, pain relieving, and soporific. I might prep my bedroom by diffusing a sedating oil, so I am set for a relaxing, restorative sleep. If that doesn't work, I choose a few new oils to give me a fresh sensory perspective. Next, I ask myself, "What am I doing?" The answer could be that I'm tensing my neck because my desk chair is too low, so I raise it and adjust my posture to be more erect. Or it could be that I haven't taken a breather—what an appropriate word. If that's the case, I do some stretching, moving, and breathing (or go for a swim in the hot springs near my cabin). I adjust my behavior as needed.

To select the oils or the blends I have on hand, I revisit my two questions: "What is really bothering me?" and "What am I doing?" Perhaps the reason I was tensing my neck muscles was the anxiety I felt about the next day or the task at hand, not the chair I was sitting in. I will choose a clary sage and lavender blend or a melissa, ylang-ylang, and spikenard blend for my sleep to soothe my anxiety. Often, personalizing my sleep oil for what I feel I need that night helps me realize there is an underlying issue I need to acknowledge and address. Maybe I need to use an oil during the day that helps me slow down, breathe deeper, and locate the source of my distractions. Being conscious of what's happening in the moment can help me, and you, transition standardized "home remedies" into customized forms of holistic self-healing. Though your process may be simpler, since you are just learning about the oils, tuning in to what your mind and body really need in the moment can make all the difference in the world.

In this chapter, I'll offer you the same tools I use to stay healthy and show you, step by step, how to build a holistic medicine cabinet of essential oils for yourself and your loved ones, including children, the elderly, and pets. I'll also provide instructions on how to prepare for the unexpected. Just like a normal medicine cabinet, your stock of essential oils will contain what you use on a regular basis (like lotions) but also what you need less often, in case of an emergency or injury (like Band-Aids). Combined with the next two chapters, which offer advice on how to buy oils and more about individual oils, this vital information will help you figure out which oils you need to always have on hand to remedy any situation, big or small, expected or unexpected.

Before we begin, here's a recap of how to use essential oils properly. Remember, when you use essential oils every day, it's important to make sure the oils are organic.

• Inhalation is the quickest way to get an essential oil's microparticles into your body and feel its effect. These microparticles are the active ingredients of all essential oils, and 70 percent of what you inhale is absorbed. Inhale essential oils in the shower, from a bowl of steam, with your slow breathing inhalations, or by anointing acupoints on your face, head, and neck.

• For local issues—like pain, injury, or congestion—target your oils at the exact location of the problem, and use a more concentrated blend. Rollerball applicators can be very helpful for muscles, because you can use the ball as a massage tool, pressing into the muscles to get your blood moving and flush out any trapped fluids.

• For a systemic issue—like stress, hot flashes, poor sleep, etc.—combine inhalation with a full-body application. Inhalation will help with changing your mind-set, and a full-body application every day slowly cues your body to adapt to the immediate stressor, by rebalancing your hormones, adjusting your body temperature, and letting your autonomic nervous system take over—the relaxation response.

• Using essential oils every day doesn't mean using the same essential oils every day. Switch it up: change your oils and routine every few days, or at least every few weeks—the same as you would with shampoo. And avoid using the same oil combination longer than three months.

• Different applications require different levels of dilution. The way you use an essential oil, and to what end, will determine whether and how much you dilute it. For example, for a tension headache, you will use 100% essential oils on the back of your neck because you are only using a couple of drops and you want the action to be very concentrated and immediate. For a relaxing body oil, you should dilute an essential oil in jojoba. The Dilution Chart in chapter 2 (page 46) provides instructions on how much or little to dilute essential oils for various applications.

Setting Up Your Medicine Cabinet

In this chapter, I offer four different options for setting up your medicine cabinet. Which option you choose is completely up to you.

Option 1 is a quick start: buying ready-made blends and products with essential oils.

Option 2 is for you if you want to swap your over-the-counter products for essential oils, using one or two oils at a time.

Option 3 is a great choice if you want to take a more thorough holistic approach and use essential oils on a daily basis, because it allows you to make your own blends.

Option 4 also offers a holistic approach but requires more time and creativity, because you'll be customizing your blends to target specific needs.

All of these options use synergistic blends of essential oils. In general, essential oils are more efficacious when combined than when used singly. The use of blends is a standard aromatherapy practice, and a recent study has shown just how beneficial that can be: when eucalyptus and tea tree oil were combined, their antimicrobial effect was almost twice as powerful than when either oil was used independently.

Option 1: Using Ready-Made Blends

This option is the quickest way for a beginner to put together a medicine cabinet of essential-oil-based remedies and personal care products. There are many ready-made blends and products available that really work. Having made my own set, I know how much easier it can be to have blends ready to go whenever you need them. Simply buy what you need from trusted aromatherapy experts, natural pharmacies or apothecaries, or health food stores. Each blend or product will come with directions for its use, and when you run out, simply purchase more! The following is a list of remedies for common conditions and the essential oils to look for in each ready-made blend or personal care product:

Allergy remedies: Look for inhalers or dropper bottles that include German chamomile, niaouli, and/or helichrysum. Test out the product first by applying the oil to a tissue, and avoid diffuser oils that trigger further irritation.

Antianxiety treatments: Look for inhalers, dropper bottles, roll-on bottles, or bath oils that include clary sage, chamomile, frankincense, lavender, mandarin, orange, rose, sandalwood, spikenard, tangerine, vetiver, and/or neroli. If an oil I haven't listed works for you, by all means find products that include it!

Antidepressants: Look for products with uplifting oils, like jasmine, ylang-ylang, lemon, lime, grapefruit, and/or bergamot, or stimulating/focusing oils, like basil, eucalyptus, peppermint, and/or pine. Also, look for the antianxiety oils to help balance your mood.

Body care: For most body care products available, there's no way of truly knowing the quality or quantity of essential oils used in them, or even in an individual bottle of oil. There's a chance you will not experience anything beyond the pleasant fragrance of the oils. Since it takes almost twenty-four hours to fully absorb an essential oil topically, when you use a shampoo, soap, or body wash that includes essential oil, you will usually rinse off all the oil in the product before your skin has had a chance to absorb it. Any effect would be the result of the scent alone (the inhalation levels are equally low). As an alternative, see chapter 2 and options 2 through 4 in this chapter for ways to make your own body oil, which will stay on your skin while it is absorbed.

Cold and flu remedies: Look for nasal sprays or inhalers that include niaouli, ravensara or eucalyptus, tea tree, spruce, pine, rosemary, fir, bay laurel, and/or lemon.

Cold sore and canker sore treatments: Look for balms that include ravensara, tea tree, niaouli, and/or myrrh.

Dental care: Look for toothpaste, toothpicks, floss, or breath fresheners that include clove, cinnamon bark, myrrh, peppermint, fennel, and/or tea tree.

Deodorants: Look for drying creams that include grapefruit, geranium, lemon, and/or lavender. Avoid alcohol-based products.

Dog care: There are many options available in pet stores and health food stores. For fear and anxiety, look for relaxing oils that include lavender, clary sage, chamomile, and/or vetiver. Always test first: let your dog smell the oil from a foot away. If they walk away or turn their head away, try another. If they face you, eyes blinking or closed (it will look like they are drinking in the scent), they come toward you, or they jump up on you, you have a winner! Never apply an oil to a dog's skin or place the oil where they can lick it off; instead, let your dog inhale it from a tissue, or put it on your hands first and then apply it lightly to the ends of the dog's fur (however, I never found this option to have worked for my dogs). Remember, their sense of smell is very evolved and that sense is unique to each dog.

Hand sanitizers: Look for gels and sprays that include thyme. Avoid alcohol-based products.

Headache remedies: Look for dropper or roll-on bottles that include peppermint, lavender, and/or helichrysum.

Indigestion relief: Look for peppermint in natural mints or in capsule form. (Colpermin and Mintec are two widely available over-the-counter brands you can buy in drugstores or online.)

Insect repellents: Look for sprays and balms that include catnip, clove, lemon eucalyptus (which the CDC recommends as an alternative to DEET), peppermint, lavender, and/or vanilla (which repels gnats).

Muscle soreness treatments: Look for diluted oils or gels that include birch, peppermint, lavender, and/or helichrysum. Avoid menthol and camphor.

PMS remedies: Look for inhalers, dropper bottles, roll-on bottles, and massage oils. For hormone balancing, look for clary sage and/or geranium; for bloating, look for cypress, lemon, geranium, birch, and/or cedarwood; for pain, see the oils under *Muscle soreness treatments* in this list; for spasms, look for products with basil, lavender, and/or chamomile (though many oils are muscle relaxers); and for mood adjustment, look at the oils under *Antidepressants* in this list.

Skin care: Look for dropper bottles, pump bottles, or creams that include carrot, helichrysum, neroli, sandalwood, jasmine, ylang-ylang, geranium, lavender, rose, clary sage, German or Roman chamomile, and/or palmarosa.

Wound healers: Look for balms that include helichrysum, myrrh, and/or lavender, or these fatty oils: arnica, Saint-John's-wort, and/or calophyllum (also known as tamanu).

Option 2: Using Single Oils and Simple Blends

The following is a list of twelve essential oils to add to your primary oils (cedarwood, lavender, lemon, peppermint, and tea tree) that create a terrific foundation for your collection. These oils are also multifunctional, easily available, user friendly, and tend to be crowd pleasers. To make it easier for you, I have paired each of these oils with the various preparations you would normally have in your medicine cabinet, along with the directions on how to use each. Feel free to use an oil by itself or dilute it in a fatty oil as directed. If you would like to use two oils together, you are creating a blend! Combine them as directed.

Acquire these additional twelve oils gradually. Instead of running out and buying them all (or filling up an online shopping cart), start with two or three oils that appeal to you. If you've purchased some of the alternate oils from chapter 1, you may already have some of the twelve, and if you are using the substitute, continue to do so here. (Also, if you own oils that aren't on this list of twelve, refer to chapter 7 for substitutions; you may not need to buy more just yet.)

TWELVE OILS FOR THE MEDICINE CABINET

Bay laurel	Grapefruit
Clary sage	Helichrysum
Clove	Pine
Eucalyptus globulus	Rosemary
Frankincense	Sandalwood
German chamomile	Vetiver

Directions for Use

Select one or two oils, dilute them if necessary (according to the Dilution Chart), and use them as directed. If you are using two oils, use equal parts of both as directed. For example, with 2 drops needed, use 1 drop of each oil; for 12 drops needed, use 6 drops of each oil.

Aftershave substitute: Lavender or lemon and lavender hydrosol; sandalwood and sandalwood hydrosol (see page 23)

Directions: Dilute 25 drops of lavender or lemon in a 4-ounce glass Boston round bottle of lavender hydrosol (you may need to remove ¼ teaspoon hydrosol from the bottle to make room for the essential oils) and pat the mixture on the skin. For sensitive skin, invest in some sandalwood and dilute 20 drops in a sandalwood hydrosol instead.

Allergy relief: Niaouli, German chamomile (as an antihistamine), helichrysum, and/or pine (for fatigue)

Directions: Use 1 or 2 drops in a bowl of hot water for inhalations and/ or cover a larger area and dilute as per a treatment oil: blend 12 drops with ½ teaspoon fatty oil in your hand and then spread the blend over the neck, chest, and throat. Avoid touching the face as much as possible. Also, use a saline neti pot to flush allergens out of the sinuses daily.

Anxiety relief: Clary sage, lavender, German chamomile, lemon, eucalyptus globulus, and/or pine (for depression)

Directions: Anoint 1 drop on the temples and place 1 drop in the palms with slow breathing inhalations. Also, dilute as per a body oil: blend 4 drops with ½ teaspoon fatty oil in your hand, rub your hands together, and spread the blend over the neck, arms, chest, legs, and lower back.

Aspirin substitute: Peppermint, helichrysum, lavender, and/or clove (clove must always be diluted for topical application)

Directions: Smooth 1 or 2 drops of peppermint on the location of acute pain or at the base of the skull for headaches. To relieve soreness around the hub of the pain, blend 2 drops of helichrysum and 10 drops of lavender with ½ teaspoon fatty oil in your hand (as per a treatment oil). Rub your hands together and then spread the blend over the area around the pain. For chronic pain, it is best to create an alternative blend; substitute 1 drop of clove for helichrysum in the dilution. (See option 4 for more on addressing pain with essential oils.)

Athlete's foot remedy: Tea tree, clove (diluted), lavender, and/or pine

Directions: Apply 4 or 5 drops to the fingertips and spread the oil along the backs of the toes of each foot in the morning and any time you change your shoes or go to the gym. Also, tap the oil onto your cotton socks or in your shoes at the end of the day.

Caffeine substitute: Peppermint, eucalyptus globulus, and/or pine

Directions: Smooth 1 or 2 drops of peppermint on the back of your neck, across your hairline. For a morning wake-up, blend 1 drop each of eucalyptus globulus and pine with ½ teaspoon fatty oil in your hand and then spread the blend over the chest and lower back, and step into the shower to breathe in the vapors.

Cleaner and room deodorizer: Lemon, clove, and/or pine (clove is not for diffusing)

Directions: Add 1 teaspoon oil to a bottle of unscented household cleanser or your own homemade cleanser (made by combining roughly 1 part white vinegar and 1 part baking soda to 2 parts water). Use 4 to 6 drops of lemon and/or pine in your diffuser as a deodorizer.

Cough expectorant: Pine and eucalyptus globulus for the flu; combine with 1 drop of helichrysum for a dry cough or asthma

Directions: Dilute as per a treatment oil by blending 12 drops with ½ teaspoon fatty oil in your hand, and then spread the blend over the neck, chest, and shoulders. Get into a shower or tub if you don't have a fever.

Deodorant: Lavender, grapefruit, or clary sage—antimicrobials easy on the skin—plus a drop of vetiver, cedarwood, frankincense, myrrh, or sandalwood to hold the scent longer

Directions: Use 1 or 2 drops in each armpit (do not use after shaving or a hot bath)

Digestive aid (for bloating or cramping): Peppermint

Directions: Inhale the oil from a tissue for nausea. Also, apply 4 drops of the oil to the abdomen in a circle and spread it over the area quickly. For abdominal cramping, follow that with a hot compress and rest with your legs up.

Diuretic: Eucalyptus globulus, grapefruit, and/or lemon

Directions: Blend 12 drops with ½ teaspoon fatty oil in your hand and then spread the blend over the legs and abdomen.

Hair care: Peppermint, rosemary, and/or clary sage

Directions: Add 1 teaspoon to an unscented shampoo and shake the bottle vigorously (this works better when the bottle is not full) and inhale as you wash. For conditioning, put 2 drops in your palm, add unscented conditioner, rub your hands together, and apply the mixture. For a hair treatment oil, blend 6 drops with ½ teaspoon jojoba oil in your hands, rub your hands together, and apply the mixture to the scalp and hair. For a styling cream, add oils to a pea-size ball of shea butter warmed by rubbing your hands together. Use fingertips to grab frizzy ends, and whole hand to smooth and polish dry patches. This is especially recommended before blow drying.

Hand sanitizer: Lavender, tea tree, and/or lemon

Directions: Place 1 or 2 drops in your damp, clean palms and smooth it over your hands. Or premix 6 drops in 2 tablespoons of aloe vera and store it in a double ziplock bag to use on the run; dispose of it after two days. Do not dilute your oils with water and keep them in a spray bottle; this will defeat the purpose.

Hot flash remedy and hormone balancing: Clary sage and/or peppermint

Directions: Dilute as per a treatment oil by blending 12 drops with

½ teaspoon fatty oil in your hand and then spread the blend over your body. Repeat the hand-blending sequence until your whole body is covered. Use this treatment twice a day. For instant temperature control, tap peppermint onto the back of your neck.

Hydrocortisone substitute (see also Wound care *and* Insect bite treatment*):* Though there aren't any natural substitutes for the synthetic topical steroid, lavender, helichrysum, and German chamomile are all anti-inflammatory, analgesic, and gentle on the skin. Pine essential oil can be added to your medicine chest for mild adrenal support, especially when diluted in anti-inflammatory olive oil or in arnica, Saint-John's-wort, or calendula-infused fatty oils. For skin conditions, herbalist Melissa Farris, who was one of the first essential oil distributors in the United States to make organic essential oils available, explains that lavender will reduce redness, swelling, and dryness; however, "neither conventional medicine nor holistic have a successful cure for eczema and psoriasis. These are better treated internally with herbal teas for purifying the blood and daily liver support (detoxifying), such as dandelion, burdock, yellow dock, and nettle." You can also find these teas fresh at your local farmers' market when the herbs are in season!

Immune support: Niaouli, tea tree, and/or bay laurel

Directions: When the immune system is taxed from lack of sleep, travel, or overdoing it, diffuse 4 to 6 drops of oil twice a day: in the morning in your bedroom and at midafternoon. You can also use tea tree in the shower by applying a drop beneath each nostril and breathing it in with the steam. Also, smooth 1 drop of bay laurel over your neck every other day to decongest your lymph nodes (apply a thin film of fatty oil over your neck first if you have sensitive skin). Support this with a daily ingestion of ginger and lemon teas. And if you feel like you are coming down with something, use *Nasal decongestant* oils and follow as directed.

Insect bite treatment: Lavender, eucalyptus globulus, clove (scabies), and/or peppermint (fleas)

Directions: Use 1 or 2 drops on the location of a bite.

Insect repellent: Peppermint, clove, eucalyptus, lemon, and/or lavender

Directions: Dilute 2 drops each of clove and peppermint, then 30 drops each of lavender, eucalyptus, and lemon in 1 tablespoon vodka and 2 tablespoons water. Shake before use and keep the blend in a spray bottle to apply it as often as needed when you are outside. Also, smooth 2 drops of essential oil blend over your hair and add a few drops on your collar, pant cuffs, and shoes.

Muscle relaxer: German chamomile, lavender, clary sage, helichrysum, and/or pine (for cold, stiff muscles)

Directions: Use 1 or 2 drops on the location of acute pain. To cover a larger area, dilute as per a treatment oil by blending 12 drops with ½ teaspoon fatty oil in your hand and then spreading the blend over the area.

Nail care: Peppermint or niaouli to stimulate the nail bed and lemon for brittle nails

Directions: Place 1 or 2 drops on your fingertip and smooth the oil over the nail beds; repeat the treatment on the other hand. Or dilute the oil in neem, walnut, and/or calophyllum oil for a cuticle treatment.

Nasal decongestant: Eucalyptus globulus (eucalyptus radiata for a hot climate), peppermint, and/or niaouli; plus, lemon and/or bay laurel

Directions: Put a drop of oil on your fingertip and place it at the opening of your nostrils. If your skin is raw, dilute 2 drops in hot water for inhalations (keep your eyes tightly shut), or put 2 drops of lemon in a bowl of hot water, soak a washcloth in the water, and use the cloth as a hot compress on blocked sinuses. Always start with eucalyptus at the first signs of a cold or the flu, and use a drop of bay laurel on swollen lymph nodes (apply a thin film of fatty oil over your neck first if you have sensitive skin).

Sleep aid: Clary sage, lavender, German chamomile, frankincense, and/or vetiver

Directions: After all other sleep preparations are complete, the lights are off, and you are in bed, use 3 to 5 drops of oil on a tissue or organic cotton wipe and hold it up to your nose. Perform twelve to fifteen slow breathing inhalations. Put the tissue aside and consciously relax your whole body, from your hands to your arms, neck, shoulders, down your back to your hips, legs, ankles, and feet. If you wake up, repeat this sequence. If you feel too awake to lie down, take a hot bath and/or drink hot milk until you get tired again. Allow for extra time for sleep when you are not sleeping straight through the night. Use a sleep mask if you are awoken by light, and always get a minimum of six hours (though eight is preferable). See the Sleep program in chapter 4 for more tips.

Sore throat or swollen glands relief: Bay laurel and/or grapefruit

Directions: Put 1 or 2 drops on your fingertips and anoint your lymph nodes/swollen glands. (Apply a thin film of fatty oil over your neck first if you have sensitive skin.)

Wound care: Lavender, helichrysum, and/or German chamomile; niaouli and/or grapefruit for varicose veins

Directions: To heal a thoroughly cleaned open wound, protect with a drop of lavender on a Band-Aid. For a healing blend, mix in your palm 2 drops each of helichrysum, lavender, and German chamomile and 1 tablespoon of the fatty oil calophyllum (tamanu) or vitamin E. To treat a burn, immediately cool the area with ice, then add 1 drop of helichrysum on a cotton ball and tap it lightly over the area.

TAKING YOUR MEDICINE CABINET ON THE ROAD

When traveling with your oils: Make a portable version of your essential oils medicine cabinet in drop-proof, 5-milliliter European dropper bottles. Keep the bottles at least halfway full and store them in the fridge in a double ziplock bag. Given their small size, these bottles will easily go through airport security, and you can just pop them into your luggage when you pack.

Option 3: Using DIY Program Blends

This option is the most cost effective. Instead of buying twelve oils or a collection of ready-made remedies, purchase four to eight individual key oils in order to make two or three blends from the following list, some of which were used in the programs in chapter 4. Whether you flip back to chapter 4 to follow a program or simply keep these blends on hand as needed, the holistic approach of using essential oils every day is simplified in these formulas (all the 100% blends go in 5-milliliter droppers):

Clear Your Chest: ¾ teaspoon fir or spruce or pine + ¼ teaspoon hyssop decumbens diluted in jojoba as per treatment oil in a 1-ounce Boston round

Clear Your Head: ¼ teaspoon eucalyptus + ¼ teaspoon rosemary + ¾ teaspoon lemon or lime

Easy Day: ½ teaspoon petitgrain + ¼ teaspoon clary sage + ¾ teaspoon lavender diluted in jojoba as per treatment oil in a 2-ounce Boston round

Focus with Calm: ¾ teaspoon lavender + ¼ teaspoon geranium + 15 drops cardamom

Relax Your Back: 64 drops lavender + 42 drops basil + 8 drops German chamomile + 8 drops peppermint diluted in jojoba as per treatment oil in a 1-ounce Boston round

Relax Your Breathing: 40 drops sandalwood + 64 drops lavender + 32 drops petitgrain + 8 drops mandarin

Shift Gears: ½ teaspoon mandarin + ½ teaspoon clary sage

Sleep Solid: ¼ teaspoon spikenard + ½ teaspoon lavender

Strengthen Your Mind: ½ teaspoon basil + 23 drops frankincense

Time Out: ½ teaspoon cypress + ½ teaspoon lavender, or 60 drops palmarosa + 4 drops peppermint + 4 drops lavender to cool off

Travel All: 26 drops litsea cubeba + 20 drops grapefruit + 32 drops cypress + 32 drops cedarwood diluted in jojoba as per body oil in a 2-ounce Boston round

Face oil: Combine 12 drops essential oils (equal parts of each oil recommended for your skin type) with 1 teaspoon rosehip seed oil, 2 teaspoons avocado oil, and 1 tablespoon jojoba oil.

Face scrub: In your palm, place 1 teaspoon scrubbing granules. Spray them with lavender, helichrysum, or neroli hydrosol until the mixture becomes the thickness of oatmeal. Apply the scrub in small circular motions and follow the lymphatic drainage massage method (from the Skin Care program, page 126).

Face mask: In your palm, place 1 teaspoon powdered clay. Spray it with hydrosol until the mixture is the thickness of yogurt (not Greek style!). Pat the mask onto your skin, avoiding the eyes. Rest with your eyes closed (and apply cold, peeled cucumber slices to your lids if you'd like).

Blemish treatment: This is a superior combination. Combine 8 drops lavender, 2 drops helichrysum, 1 drop German chamomile (anti-inflammatory), and 6 drops tea tree (antimicrobial). Apply it with a cotton swab.

Option 4: Using DIY Customized Blends

This option is perfect if you want to focus on pain relief, find a healthy way to lose weight, or feel calm and connected (especially during pregnancy and childbirth, and postpartum, for all you mamas out there). Whether you use your new blends and techniques every day or use them at key instances when you need them most, they will fit your needs at the moment.

Customized blends create a more targeted form of relief. Everyone has their own unique health and lifestyle challenges. When you choose not to follow a cookie-cutter plan, you give yourself the opportunity to build habits that match your body and mind. For this holistic approach, the positive results will be their own reward.

Pain Relief

Chronic pain is a huge area of study all on its own, but it's important to remember that when we suppress pain, we block much-needed warnings from our bodies. All of my clients with back pain typically recount, "I just twisted a little bit when I bent forward and I couldn't move for a week, and I am still living with that pain." When a seemingly simple movement triggers a disabling injury, it is often an indication that the warning signs from the pain centers of the brain are not getting through to our consciousness.

Without body awareness of signs and symptoms, we may not know a major injury is brewing. We need to stay in touch with our bodies, especially if we sit for long periods of time at a computer, which is hard on the back, neck, and shoulders and even the arms and hands. Pain is exacerbated by excess tension, which in turn leads to more pain. Essential oil rituals, like Relax Your Body Time (page 115), keep us in touch and ease discomfort.

The following blends help remedy the types of pain people tend to feel when life (and work) starts to resemble sitting in an airplane seat for hours every day:

• *Arthritis:* For the best anti-inflammatory and cooling, relaxing pain relief, mix and dilute this blend as per a treatment oil in a 1-ounce Boston round: ¾ teaspoon lavender + 6 drops German chamomile + 8 drops helichrysum + 8 drops peppermint. Fill with jojoba, cap, and tip the bottle up and down until fully mixed. Apply where it hurts.

• *Facial or nerve pain:* For calming oils that reduce redness, mix and dilute this blend as per a facial oil in a 1-ounce Boston round: ¼ teaspoon palmarosa (especially good for TMJ) + 3 drops German chamomile + 3 drops lavender. Fill with jojoba, cap, and tip the bottle up and down until fully mixed. Starting at the ears, apply along the jawline.

• *Hangover:* To support an overtaxed liver as well as relieve headache symptoms, mix and dilute this blend as per a treatment oil in a 1-ounce Boston round: 15 drops peppermint + 4 drops helichrysum + ¾ teaspoon lemon. Fill with jojoba, cap, and tip the bottle up and down until fully mixed. Apply the mixture to the neck, shoulders, and temples. Do slow breathing inhalations with 4 or 5 drops of this blend in your palms for nausea.

• *Headache:* For on-the-spot relief, apply a drop of 100% peppermint, lavender, or eucalyptus to the base of your skull. If a headache accompanies an earache, apply a drop to the acupoint at the base of the thumb, in between the thumb and first finger, and to the temples (lavender or eucalyptus only; always keep peppermint away from your eyes).

• *Localized muscle pain:* Combine analgesics and anti-inflammatories, such as 8 drops peppermint or 8 drops helichrysum, with 1 scant teaspoon of your combination of muscle-relaxing vetiver, lavender, and/or basil, since they warm the muscles and move the blood through the area constricted by pain. Mix and dilute this blend as per a treatment oil in a 1-ounce Boston round. Fill with jojoba, cap, and tip the bottle up and down until fully mixed. Apply directly to the painful area two or three times a day.

• *Pain worse during damp weather:* Add 5 to 10 extra drops of litsea cubeba, birch, or eucalyptus to your muscle pain treatment oil.

• *PMS or menstrual cramps:* Combine ½ teaspoon lavender + 10 drops basil + ¼ teaspoon clary sage + 6 drops helichrysum. Mix and dilute this blend as per a treatment oil in a 1-ounce Boston round. Fill with jojoba, cap, and tip the bottle up and down until fully mixed. Apply it to the lower back and abdomen (follow this with a heating pad). For bloating, add a few drops of peppermint on top of the treatment oil.

Weight Loss

Weight loss is about relearning what taking good care of yourself feels like. The more ways you can indulge and reward yourself without reaching for calorie-rich, nutrition-poor foods, the more your body can change. When you cut down calories, your body learns how to get by with less, which can make the process of losing weight difficult and slow. Essential oils can be a useful aid to help you succeed at staying healthy while losing weight. Here's how essential oils can help:

• *To reduce cravings:* Have you ever noticed that when you get less than six hours of sleep your body goes into a prediabetic state and ups your sugar cravings? It is of utmost importance to keep your blood sugar balanced, reduce your anxiety and irritability, get good quality sleep, and have good digestion in order to control your cravings. To balance your blood sugar with essential oils, slice half a lemon into four pieces and squeeze the slices into a tall glass, then add the squeezed rinds and fill the glass with water. Refill this glass with water three more times and drink from it throughout your day.

• *To aid digestion:* When bloating and pain from IBS are distressing, it can be hard to stay focused on your diet. Moreover, if you aren't absorbing the nutrients from the healthy foods you're eating, your cravings are amped up—or, worse, your appetite drops until all of a sudden you're ravenous and can't make wise choices, or you eat too late at night, which in turn disturbs your sleep. To aid digestion most effectively, you really need to take peppermint internally. To do that safely, without the risk of developing or exacerbating reflux or irritating the mucous membranes of your digestive tract, I recommend taking peppermint in capsule form (page 151) in conjunction with an abdominal massage using 4 drops of peppermint essential oil spread over the abdomen. If this irritates your skin, follow with a light fatty oil, like grape seed. Apply a heating pad to deepen the relaxing effects, relax cramping, and ease distress. If you are experiencing painful cramping, add 2 drops of helichrysum on top of the peppermint and then follow with the fatty oil and a hot compress or heating pad. Abdominal massage can also help release emotional distress. Lightly smooth your hands clockwise over your abdomen as you take a stress-relieving break. Also, include probiotic foods (yogurt, kefir, fermented live foods) to aid digestion and support intestinal flora.

• *To reduce fluid retention and cellulite:* Diuretic essential oils help move fluids trapped in tissue due to sitting at a computer too long or a lack of exercise. Starting a new exercise program while changing your diet could be overwhelming. Instead, make a blend of 5 drops fennel + ¼ teaspoon cypress + ½ teaspoon grapefruit + ¼ teaspoon cedarwood + 10 drops birch and transfer to a 2-ounce Boston round. Mix and dilute this blend as per a treatment oil. Fill with grape seed oil, cap, and tip the bottle up and down until fully mixed.

Apply it to your ankles, legs, and hips in the morning using the After Your Shower ritual (page 59). When you have time at the end of the day, apply it after dry-brushing your skin and using the alternating water temperature technique outlined in For the Total Spa Experience (page 70). Your return to exercise can be as simple as a daily practice of walking five thousand steps coupled with How to Get a Mini Workout Anytime (page 66) several times a day.

• *To reduce irritability or mood swings:* As your body detoxes, your emotions can too. The quickest way to shift your mood is with slow breathing inhalations from a few drops of a 100% essential oil in your palms. Don't wait until your food cravings take over. Instead, choose from or make a simple blend with clary sage, lavender, geranium, sandalwood, neroli, rose, and/or any oil that helps you feel nurtured and calm. Place a drop on your perfume points, or in your palm for slow breathing inhalations, or in a glass by your computer to swirl and inhale, as in For a Quick Desk Break ritual (page 60).

Pregnancy, Childbirth, and Postpartum

When you're pregnant, everything that you apply to your skin or inhale can make its way to your baby in utero. It's important to consider the baby first and to err on the side of caution, even when it comes to using essential oils. So I need to note that you should not use essential oils during the first trimester of pregnancy. There are many essential oils that are beneficial to use during the second and third trimesters. In general, pregnant or nursing mothers should dilute oils at 1% (see the Dilution Chart, page 46) and choose flowers and citrus oils over spice oils. But just as it's impossible to predict the weird food cravings you might experience, it's also impossible to predict what oils will help you feel good when you're pregnant. Try out the oils that are recommended and see which ones make you feel soothed, relaxed, calm, and taken care of. For nausea or morning sickness, inhale a little peppermint and see if that works for you. If not, try the dried herbs themselves: make a chamomile and peppermint tea or an iced version of chamomile tea with sprigs of fresh mint.

Once you know which oils are right for you, make your own blend of two or three oils and dilute them in jojoba oil (see the Dilution Chart). Use your pregnancy body oil after showering to keep your skin moist. You can also use it to moisturize anytime and in your hair to keep it glossy. For minimal stretch marks, follow the oil treatment with shea butter as often as needed for your skin to feel supple and soothed. You can also use coconut oil or an unscented body balm with organic beeswax, shea butter, and coconut oil. If there are oils you like to inhale that soothe your mind, make a second blend, diluted as per a pregnancy body oil in a 10-milliliter roller bottle to take with you so you can roll it on your temples and other acupoints as you choose.

Your basic guideline for using oils throughout your pregnancy is

• *Dilute your oils more.* Switch from targeted treatments to dilution levels also recommended for children (1%). Use essential oils undiluted for inhalation only.

• *Smell before you apply,* so you can anticipate your reactions. I have known pregnant women who lose their lunch after inhaling lavender, a scent they loved before conception. There's no way to know how you will react ahead of time.

• *Relax.* The essential oils that are right for you are the ones that help you relax, take it slow, listen to your body, and breathe comfortably.

• *Take baths.* Put 4 drops under the spigot and swish to disperse once you are in the tub. Put a bath pillow or rolled-up towel under your neck, lie back, and let your mind wander, or focus on your breathing to calm your worries.

OILS FOR PREGNANCY, CHILDBIRTH, AND POSTPARTUM

Here are the safest, most commonly used oils for use during and after pregnancy:

• *First trimester:* Avoid essential oils during your first trimester.

• *Second and third trimesters:* Lavender, neroli, rose otto, ylang-ylang, geranium, mandarin, German chamomile, petitgrain, sandalwood, grapefruit, lemon, sweet orange (although not exclusively and not every day), cypress, tea tree, eucalyptus, frankincense, and benzoin. Bergamot can be very uplifting, by itself as an inhalant from a tissue or from your palms (even if you aren't pregnant!), or dilute with jojoba, palmarosa, and a tiny drop of patchouli; mix these four oils first in a glass to make sure you aren't including too much patchouli. This is one of the most emotionally soothing blends.

OILS TO AVOID

I recommend avoiding anise, basil (except 1 drop during childbirth), birch, eucalyptus, camphor, caraway, carrot, cinnamon, clove, cumin, fennel, hyssop, lemongrass, lemon myrtle, litsea cubeba, myrrh, niaouli, nutmeg, oregano, rosemary, savory, thyme, and wintergreen. Reserve peppermint for light inhalation to alleviate nausea during pregnancy, but do not use it during childbirth, lactation, or with children under five.

All the oils listed should also not be used with young children. Children under five should *not* be exposed to eucalyptus, fennel, peppermint, and rosemary because these are all very strong essential oils. In general, use your common sense. *Avoid* using essential oils on or near infants, and keep in mind that young children (over the age of one) need a more diluted product and are always treated gently with essential oils, as with everything else.

PREGNANCY SYMPTOMS AND OILS TO TREAT THEM

Nausea: Breathing in from the bottle or a tissue, perform slow breathing inhalations with peppermint (do not use topically).

Lack of sleep: Place a drop of neroli, rose, or sandalwood in your palms for slow breathing inhalations, or for a more cost-effective use of these precious oils, blend together 2 drops of each and add to a 10-milliliter European dropper or roll-on bottle, fill with jojoba oil, label, and store. Apply the blend to a tissue for slow breathing inhalations as often as needed throughout the night, while in bed.

Lower back pain: Combine 5 drops of neroli with 20 drops of sandalwood and dilute the mixture in jojoba as per a pregnancy body oil on the Dilution Chart (page 46). Apply the blend to your lower back and hips.

Cold, flu, and sinus congestion: Inhale drops of 100% tea tree oil from a tissue five times a day.

Labor pains: Lavender is the most commonly used oil for slowing down contractions—if you want that! Clary sage should help get them started. Diffuse these in the delivery room for ten to fifteen minutes at a time. A blend of 1 drop each of basil, myrrh, and jasmine can be a stimulating back rub, diluted as per a massage oil. Or choose 1 drop each of rose, lavender, and ylang-ylang, diluted as per a massage oil, which can help relax your neck, shoulders, and back in between contractions, hopefully lifting your mood! Bring some organic cotton clothes to soak with oils for inhalations (as an alternative to diffusing), like lavender to calm or lemon to stimulate, and use some tea tree to swab down the bathroom and sanitize your area.

Postpartum stress: For emotional stress, dilute equal parts clary sage and geranium in jojoba oil as per a massage oil for a face, neck, or shoulder massage, or put 1 drop of each on a tissue and inhale, and book a massage!

Take Care

Each time I feel something is out of whack with my body or mind, I return to holistic self-care. By doing so, I try to learn as much as I can about the underlying issues that caused me to feel out of sorts. This not only ensures immediate relief but also can help me prevent an injury or illness from recurring in the future.

What I've learned so many times while dealing with my health challenges is that the sooner I realize something is wrong, the more effective this gentle, natural approach will be. I've included tips and instructions about self-awareness and healing that I've learned over the years so that you too can take a proactive approach to speed your healing and stay well.

Breathing deeper, relaxing your neck, or taking a break to rest changes everything where your body's healing process is concerned. You simply won't find relief when you ignore or attempt to turn off your body's feedback mechanisms. So many people sacrifice health and well-being to meet a deadline, be a perfectionist, or get everything done, myself included. I see this behavior repeatedly in my practice. For example, my client Marsha was so dedicated to her job, which required constant travel, that she didn't realize she was pregnant until she miscarried late in her first trimester. Another client Mallory gave up tennis, a sport she adored, simply because she hadn't given her most recent injury time to heal, but after working with me, she was able to return to the court pain-free. Or Joanne, who was constantly in pain at work because her clothes were too tight (I kid you not). I once had a woman visit me with a sore neck because her prescription glasses desperately needed to be updated. Sometimes the answers to our physical and mental ailments are so simple—but we're too busy being busy to ask the questions.

Now that you've learned how to build a medicine cabinet of essential oils, it's time to go shopping! In the next chapter, I'll share everything you need to know about buying quality essential oils.

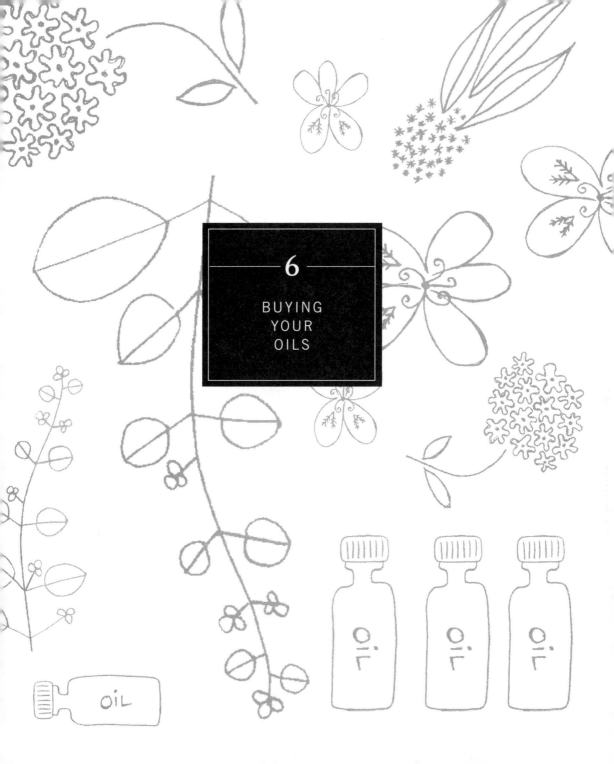

6

BUYING
YOUR
OILS

I was first introduced to essential oils through massage, but it was water that invited me into my work with oils. After my first transformative session, my aromatherapist stressed the benefit of a daily program of hydrotherapy. Baths were a great place for me to start. Each bath was different depending on what oils I added to it. As I continued to experiment, the blend of aromatics thoroughly shaped my mood and eased my body's stresses. It was a very spontaneous process.

Admittedly, early on I made mistakes. One time I applied two of the hottest oils, ginger and lemongrass, directly to my skin. Ouch, that stung! I also quickly figured out that you shouldn't add oils to the bathwater until you are already in the tub or they will attach to your body in all the wrong places. I also learned that baths weren't just for bedtime (although to help you sleep, baths are definitely supreme). Eventually, I switched to taking short baths in the morning, instead of showers, to help me wake up using my new elixirs. I looked forward to the experience every morning as my alarm went off.

Of course, it was no coincidence that I began with baths since water is familiar to dancers. Those of us who are passionate about dance spend hours soaking, steaming, and heating our muscles to stay on our feet. Ultimately, dance is about fluidity. A mountain river fed by melting snow can be strong, gentle, or weak, but it's perpetual. Dancing well is similar; regardless of how fast or slow you may be moving, it's about keeping the muscles engaged so that a flow of movement continues.

When you bring new oils into your home, you are welcoming in a similar flow of energy. Think about all the plants that go into a single bottle of essential oil. Imagine the hundreds of plants that have gone into the oil as its microparticles flow freely into your body with each inhale of the oil or when you apply it to your skin. As the oils travel through your body, you are helping your blood to circulate better, bringing the energy from the plants to your mind and muscles.

When you bring home essential oils, you are bringing home entire fields of healers. This is where your therapeutic results begin. Before you purchase an oil, visualize how you want to feel or how you want to smell. Do a little research about the plant the oil comes from. Visualize the terrain of its natural environment. The more your imagination and mind get involved, the fuller your meditative slow breathing inhalations will be. Give yourself a moment to put aside all rationale and logic. Start with the notion that you are bringing a vibrant piece of nature into your body and your mind.

Finding Quality Essential Oils

I bought my first oils from my aromatherapist directly, which is an easy way to ensure quality. When I started working with oils and ran out of something that I needed in a pinch, I would get a replacement at my local health food store or from a few herbal boutiques in lower Manhattan. There were only a few oils available at that time and no organic aromatics at all.

When I first started looking for oils to purchase, the practice of adding synthetic room fragrance to a bowl of multicolored potpourri was big. It was hard to distinguish between synthetic and essential oils, especially because the products were all displayed together.

Today, it can still be difficult to find authentic oils, especially when 98 percent of the oils that end up in the products we bring into our homes are not in their authentic state. Since the availability (and cost) of essential oils varies throughout the year, as a professional, I have to work with a few different suppliers. Even then, I am always on the lookout for better-quality oils. For example, I worked my way through at least ten different sources for vetiver before finally settling on two great distributors.

In this chapter, I'll streamline what I've learned in the past twenty years about buying essential oils. My advice will help you find the best quality oils your budget can manage, both online and in stores.

Does Synthetic Mean Chemical?

A lot of people want to avoid "chemicals," but those people are using the wrong term. Everything in the world is a chemical; elements, such as carbon, oxygen, and hydrogen, combine to make chemicals. Even water is a chemical, because it's made of two hydrogen atoms and one oxygen atom.

However, what you should be concerned about is whether the chemical is biosynthetic or synthetic. "Biosynthetic" means that the substance is made in nature—like essential oils. This is good. Anything "synthetic" is manmade (including ingredients that are added to make essential oils cheaper). People who say they're avoiding chemicals are really trying to avoid synthetic chemicals, because these substances and ingredients can be more harmful than their natural counterparts.

When you buy essential oils, the question to ask the salesperson is "Does this product contain synthetic ingredients or has it been synthetically altered or diluted?" If you're still not sure, your nose can help. Smell a sample. When a scent is faint or is more like perfume than a plant substance, or when you don't see basic information on the label, consider finding another source. The important thing is to buy organic oils. You may never know if an oil has been diluted with other organic oils, but in the long run the extra cost will be worth it, because the oils will still be more potent, more effective, more breathable, and free of added toxic substances.

Therapeutic Grade vs. Commercial Grade

If a distributor or seller says their oils are "therapeutic grade," that's a marketing term only. There's no third-party regulation—the manufacturer, distributor, and seller don't have to meet any requirements or standards to make this claim.

"Commercial grade" is a different term assigned to products by distributors. However, stay clear of commercial-grade essential oils. These products are used to create perfumes, scented candles, car fragrances, candy, cleaning products, soft drinks, laundry products, and beauty products, to name just a few. You *do not* want to purchase commercial-grade essential oils, because these have been standardized, primarily so the smells and flavors are consistent and match what the general consumer expects. This type of standardization correlates to adulteration, loss of potency, and synthetic and ultimately toxic ingredients.

Remember, true essential oils are not consistent. If you ever shop somewhere that claims to stock different "grades" of essential oil products, ask what the differences are. The answer should always be transparent. And if it's not, don't shop there!

What Does "Certified Organic" Mean? What About "Wild-Crafted"?

Organic farming requires practices that are important for our environment and restricts the use of synthetic pesticides and GMOs. Organic farming shows a commitment to, and supports, an agricultural system that is far preferable to conventional farming—every acre of farmland reserved for organic farming is an acre of land based on sustainability and saved from the use of harmful chemicals.

If you buy conventional oils, you have no way of knowing how much pesticide still resides in the oils, or how those oils have been obtained or treated after the initial distillation. When you buy organic essential oils, you avoid synthetic pesticides and alterations. And wouldn't you rather use the oil from a plant that has fought off bugs and diseases all on its own? After all, you want that oil to do the same for you. Buy organic.

Wild-crafted essential oils are harvested from uncultivated plants found in their natural, or "wild" habitat, like *Litsea cubeba* (also known as may chang) from China or *Santalum album* (sandalwood) from India. Since these plants don't require acres of farmland (and possible water subsidies), wild-crafted oils can be an excellent sustainable. The whole plants and roots are usually left in place while only the leaves, fruit, or flowers are collected (although Indian sandalwood is not adequately protected and is now endangered). Medicinally, since these plants draw from a broader base of genetic material and can have a more complex structure than plants that have been cloned or genetically engineered, the therapeutic impact of these plants is greater. In the aromatherapy community, wild-crafted is a preferred type of oil. However, because we only know that these oils come from plants picked in the wild, we cannot trace the path of the product from seed to bottle, unlike organic plants, which have been cultivated by farmers and extracted by distillers who must adhere to standards and regulations and submit documents.

That said, I use wild-crafted oils in my products in combination with certified organics, and you can do this too if you have the option when purchasing. U.S. regulations on organic products that have the USDA certified seal are as follows: "USDA certified" means 95% of the product must be organic; "100% organic" means the product is 100% organic. However, if you see products labeled "made with organic," they are only required to be 70% organic, so look for the USDA seal (see https://www.ams.usda.gov/).

Shopping at a Store

Now that you have read the previous chapters and figured out what oils you want to buy, the first step is to visit a health food store, a yoga studio, an herbal pharmacy, or a wellness apothecary that carries organic essential oils and get to the business of smelling. The quality of oils you find in a store may vary. Often essential oils haven't been stored properly and may have lost potency just from being on the shelf too long. In general, I think it's preferable to purchase essential oils online, especially citrus oils, which have a short shelf life and are best refrigerated. However, when you are first experimenting with oils, it's great to visit a store so you can smell and test out different oils. Notice your reactions as you inhale, because these can be memorable moments. You might discover that you absolutely adore grapefruit essential oil in the health section at your neighborhood Whole Foods, which you would have never realized shopping online. Have fun!

Use tissues to smell the aroma and tap out a few drops of each oil you want to test so you can really inhale the entire scent. Remember, the first rule of shopping for aromatics is to not smell directly from the bottle because you will miss out on the full shape of the scent. You know what to do: slow breathing inhalations, waving the tissue back and forth under your nose. Take note of which oils make you feel that sense of "Gah, I love this!" Which oil do you want to smell again? Let your senses inform your mind.

The second rule of shopping is to remember that you get what you pay for, especially with lavender and flower oils. Like a good bottle of wine, these oils are complex and unique. Lavender has more than one hundred chemical constituents! You will enjoy a quality bottle much more than the lowest-cost one available.

The same is true for all organic oils; these might be slightly more costly, but they are totally worth the extra money. The less expensive, "budget-friendly" oils are made affordable by diluting and adulterating what nature has already perfected. Be sure to buy organic citrus oils because these are cold-pressed straight from the peel and do not contain the pesticides that nonorganic oils do.

Shopping Online

Here are a few things to keep in mind when searching for a reputable website for essential oils:

• *One site is enough.* The best way to buy oils is to find one website that works for you and buy all your oils from that company. It makes it easier when you need more, and you will know what to expect when you purchase them.

• *Quality is worth every penny.* Look for sites that sell mostly, if not all, organic oils and that list the name, the Latin botanical name, the country of origin, and the specific plant part used to produce the oil. If the website sells synthetic products like thickeners, emulsifiers, fragrance oils, or preservatives, stay away; these sites are geared toward small skin care companies, not general consumers. Also, it's best to avoid large herbal online supermarkets or clearinghouses, because these outlets don't have as much knowledge about oils—or the quality of products—as smaller, more reputable vendors.

• *Aromatherapy websites are the best.* Purchasing oils directly from an experienced aromatherapist almost always guarantees quality. If the aromatherapist has published some articles in journals or on professional websites, or has an accredited school, that's all the better.

• *Get on the phone.* One of the best ways to learn about the quality of a company's oils is to talk with a knowledgeable seller. Personally, I have always preferred to buy my oils from a professional who is happy to provide the answers I need about the oils and sends the products quickly. Some great questions to ask are "Do you work directly with the grower and/or distiller?" "Do you have your own testing procedures to monitor the quality of your oils?" "Are there batch numbers on the bottles?" "How do you store your essential oils?" and "How do you make sure your business is sustainable?"

• *Build a relationship.* Once you find the right supplier, you will be rewarded by buying oils from someone you can truly trust, which makes every purchase even more exciting. Also, if the producer or aromatherapist is out of the office visiting the South of France every summer for the lavender harvest, that's a good sign!

Another aspect of buying online that causes confusion is the difference between buying extracts (derived by soaking the plant in grain alcohol) and essential oils (which are obtained through distillation or cold-pressing). Extracts and essential oils from the same plant do not necessarily have the same therapeutic properties, and extracts will be less concentrated. Though extracts have important therapeutic applications, you don't want to get your apples mixed up with your oranges. An easy way to tell the difference is that extracts are water-soluble—they dissolve in water—whereas essential oils are not. Essential oils will bead up on the surface of water. In order to be sure you are buying an essential oil, the label should very clearly state "essential oil." Extracts and even plant essences don't offer the same potency or the same benefits as true essential oils.

Storing Essential Oils

For optimal results, essential oils should be kept at cooler temperatures, less than 80 degrees Fahrenheit. On a hot day, it's useful to keep your oils close to an air-conditioner or in the coolest place in your home, like a low cabinet in a cool room since cool air remains closer to the ground. It's also okay to store essential oils in the refrigerator (which lengthens shelf life). However, essential oils need to be at room temperature in order for you to receive the full experience of the aroma. This is especially true when you are combining essential oils in a therapeutic blend or creating a brand-new blend.

Once you open an essential oil, it will retain its maximum potency for about a year, or two years if you keep it refrigerated. You want your oils to be potent for therapeutic purposes.

In general, when used purely as scents, essential oils can get better with age but will lose some potency. It's smart to always buy the oils for your therapeutic blends in small amounts so you can keep buying fresh stock. Essential oils that you have had for longer than two years are better suited for beautiful personalized perfumes, scented body care, and room deodorizers. All essential oils oxidize over time, which will change their chemistry gradually. This can affect the sensitivity you have to the oil. For example, the conifer oils (pine, spruce, fir, balsam) can be irritating to the skin if they have been stored for more than a few years. On the other hand, the scent of an oil can get richer over time. The only oils that "go bad" are the citrus oils, which *must* be stored in the refrigerator. I like to move my oils along a chain of command as each ripens and gets older, using them in therapeutics, then in perfumery, then in cleaning applications, and ultimately as pest repellents.

In addition to temperature and time, essential oil potency is affected by light. If your oils are not in the fridge, always store them away from light or heat. If you have a room that never gets direct sunlight, that would be perfect. But don't put your oils away like some souvenir you will only want to look at five years from now! Don't deny yourself the wonderful benefit of essential oils; keep your cache readily available. Buying essential oils in 5-milliliter European dropper bottles is a good way to store them, because there is very little air in the bottle, which means there will be less oxidation. Another way to prevent oxidation is to keep your bottles full. For example, if you decide to purchase a 4-ounce bottle of lavender and decant half to a smaller 2-ounce Boston round bottle after you are halfway through, your lavender will be better preserved overall.

If you are using blends every day, you will to want to keep your key oils and blends in your bathroom, kitchen, or bedroom. Here's where the dark glass bottles come in handy—blocking the light while the bottles sit on the edge of your sink or shelf. Essential oils eat through rubber, so don't bother getting bottles for your blends that have rubber droppers. And never store undiluted essential oils in plastic.

Your hydrosols need to go in the fridge too, because hydrosols (unlike 100% essential oils) will gather bacteria. And while you are at it, put all your fatty oils in the fridge. All fatty oils will eventually go rancid from oxidation, except jojoba, meadowfoam seed, and fractionated coconut oil (since this oil has been processed, even if originally organically sourced, it will never have the seal). If you discover a rancid fatty oil in your collection, get rid of it! Rancid oils are not healthy for you and should be disposed of.

Safety Is Simple

Before using a new essential oil, read about it in chapter 7, where I include specific safety recommendations and caveats on combinations. For everyone, I like to share the following basic safety tips:

Immediately remove any irritating blend, dilution, or 100% essential oil or oil applied by mistake. Do not use water or a hot towel to remove the oil, because this will accelerate its action and spread it further. The least irritating option is to remove the unwanted oil by diluting it on your skin with a fatty oil, like olive or grape seed oil, and wipe everything off at once.

Immediately discontinue use and remove the essential oil if you are having an allergic reaction, where your skin becomes inflamed and red or has raised bumps. Wash the area thoroughly with soap and then rinse with cool water. An allergic reaction is extremely rare, especially with organic essential oils, though it can be triggered by an interaction with some medications. Consult your doctor before using essential oils if you are on medication. Also, if you have a serious or chronic medical condition, it's best to discuss the use of essential oils with your doctor before starting to use them.

Immediately discontinue use and remove a commercial product that contains essential oil if you are having an allergic reaction. In this case the allergy could be due to the preservatives, perfume, or foaming agent, not the essential oil. Once the reaction has subsided, you may test out the essential oil on its own by applying a couple of drops on the crook of your elbow and waiting thirty-six hours to see if you have any reaction.

Keep essential oils out of your eyes and ears. Keep essential oils at least an inch away from your eyes and the inside of your ears, especially strong, highly volatile oils, like peppermint. If you mistakenly do get an essential oil in your eye, use olive oil or another fatty oil to remove it, like this: Soak a clean cloth in the fatty oil and gently wipe your eyelid and the outside corner of your eye. As you blink, the fatty oil will flush the eye and then you can gently wipe away the oil with a clean cotton pad, the way you wipe off your makeup. If some essential oil remains, flush your eye with warm water. If you want to put an essential oil in your ear, use the oil in a 2% dilution and put 1 drop of the dilution on a cotton ball first, then place the cotton ball only at the opening of your ear.

Consult your doctor if you have existing medical conditions. Some essential oils (like rosemary) can be contraindicated for high blood pressure and some may have negative interactions when combined with specific prescription medications, especially after surgery or in conjunction with chemotherapy. And again, if you have a serious or chronic medical condition, it's best to discuss the use of essential oils with your doctor.

Watch the sun. As mentioned previously, some essential oils—including all citrus oils (grapefruit, lemon, lime, orange, mandarin, tangerine, bergamot) and coriander, as well as ginger (which is not discussed in detail in this book)—are photosensitizing and can lead to sun damage if applied topically.

Dilute skin-sensitive oils. Of the oils I cover in chapter 7, the most sensitizing oils, when applied topically, include birch, clove, may chang, and melissa. When used topically, consider lowering the percentage of the dilution more than I recommend, if you have sensitive skin. Remember, before trying any new oil, always test the 100% oil in the crook of your elbow. Thyme, thymol, oregano, cinnamon bark, wintergreen, and savory are also skin irritants that need to be highly diluted or avoided for topical use altogether.

Always avoid . . . As you continue your explorations beyond this book, you may encounter some oils that are not recommended—some are strong irritants; some are neurotoxic. The primary offenders are pennyroyal, camphor, cinnamon leaf, hyssop officinalis (however, hyssop decumbens is safe to use), sage, mugwort, and thuja.

This concludes all the basics you need in order to buy, blend, apply, and enjoy your oils! I am so excited for you. Chapter 7 is your easy reference to all the oils I have preapproved for you.

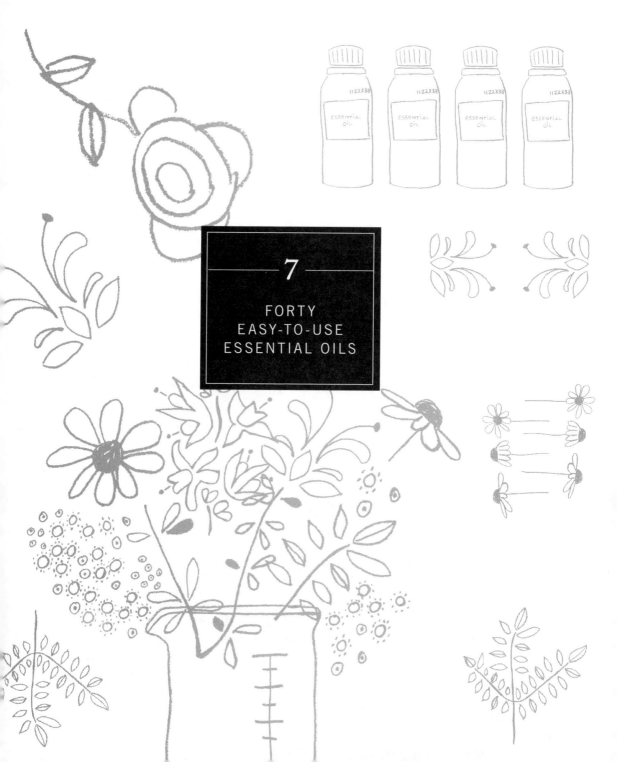

7

FORTY
EASY-TO-USE
ESSENTIAL OILS

I have spent the better part of this book providing different ways to bring essential oils into your daily life. This chapter will give you a more in-depth look at individual oils: what each essential oil does, how it is used, and what, if any, safety concerns that oil has. In choosing these oils, I wanted you to feel confident using each one and have no trouble buying them (though weather and farming issues can limit supply at certain times of the year). I chose the oils from the more than four hundred oils produced that are the easiest and safest to use, preferring oils that don't irritate your skin or require expertise to apply. I have included a few special safety precautions with oils that are just too beautiful and beneficial to pass up, like melissa and birch. It's a good idea to always read the safety instructions. I'm sure you will have your favorite, so don't feel you have to memorize the information for all forty oils. Rather, this chapter is a reference you can come back to as needed.

When you have a new issue to address or you are looking for a fresh approach to using essential oils every day, this chapter will be an invaluable resource, allowing you to delve deeper into an individual oil that you're interested in. Sometimes you may read about a specific oil in a magazine or online. Perhaps a salesperson tells you something about an essential oil that totally surprises you. The ages-old knowledge about essential oils is only beginning to be updated, by scientists, practitioners, and professionals like myself. Because of that, sources about essential oils are as likely to be incorrect as correct. Therefore, it's best to double-check what you hear, either by using the resources in this book (and specifically in this chapter) or by discussing the information with a professional in the industry.

There is so much to know about each essential oil. In the glossary that follows, I've tried to be comprehensive and concise. Each entry for a common essential oil includes information on where it comes from geographically (*source*), what part of the plant is used (*distilled from* or *cold-pressed from*), its *attributes* (color and aroma), and any *safety* precautions and *recommendations*.

ONE LAST WORD ABOUT SAFETY

In chapter 6, I provided general guidelines on how to use each oil to avoid skin irritations or negative interactions with prescription medications and over-the-counter drugs. In this chapter, I go a little bit further. For example, some oils are best used short-term, because their effects change when the oils are applied frequently. Similarly, the oils that are not safe for use by pregnant women are also not safe to use during lactation or the early life of a baby (up to two years old). Even more important, some oils that can be useful during childbirth should be avoided during the earlier stages of pregnancy, because these oils can stimulate contractions (which no one wants earlier than nature intended!). In general, it's smart to test any new oil first in the crook of your elbow to see if your skin reacts—even if that oil is listed as "safe for all purposes"—because everyone is different.

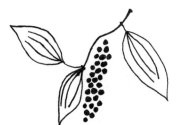

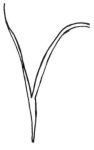

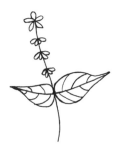

BASIL LINALOOL, SWEET (*Ocimum basilicum*)
Source: France, Italy, Egypt, Hungary, Bulgaria, United States
Distilled from: Leaves and flowering tops of the plant
Attributes: A clear, watery oil that smells strongly spicy, sometimes like licorice, sometimes like root beer. The essential oil is close to the aroma of the herb. It can be used as a top note for a spicy, earthy personal scent.
Safety: Use a small amount in your essential oil blend and dilute in a fatty oil. It is not for prolonged use or for use during pregnancy. Do not select the *ocimum gratissimum L.* variety.
Recommendations: *With its warming, anti-inflammatory, antidepressant, digestive, muscle-relaxing, adrenal-stimulating, and decongesting properties,* this versatile oil can ease aches and pains (apply it to the lower back for menstrual and back pain, on feet for gout), help you get over a cold or the flu, and bring you to a better state of mind. If you are feeling depleted or losing motivation, diffuse this oil two times a day (for short-term use) to help you get back on track. It can also be used in meditation, to restore confidence.

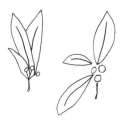

BAY LAUREL (*Laurus nobilis L.*)
Source: Croatia, Bosnia, Italy, France
Distilled from: Leaves and sometimes berries
Attributes: A clear, watery oil that smells spicy but sweet and so strong that when you stand next to the tree, you can feel the vapors in your breathing passages. The oil can be used as a top note for a refreshingly spicy personal scent.

Safety: Test it in the crook of your elbow. If the oil irritates your skin, use in cold and flu blends for inhalation only. If it does not, you can apply a drop topically for short-term use or dilute in a fatty oil. Keep away from children under one year old.

Recommendations: *With its expectorant, antimicrobial, and anti-infectious properties,* this oil also aids digestion. Diffuse it or apply it to the skin directly over the lymph nodes (the glands in your neck, armpits, and joints) if you have a sore throat or feel you are coming down with something, especially after travel. Or pair it with another strong decongestant, like eucalyptus and/or lemon, to give yourself a fighting chance to stay well.

ABOUT ABSOLUTES

Some flowers do not yield enough essential oils per bud when distilled. Instead, the oil from the flowers is extracted by using a solvent (which ranges from a harsh petrochemical to a biosynthetic for organic absolutes) and then goes through a second process to remove the solvent. The pure essence left behind is called an absolute, which is used primarily in perfumery and is not as useful for therapeutic blends (organic absolutes can be used therapeutically whereas nonorganics may be laced with toxic solvents). However, you will notice a few absolute oils in this glossary because there are several popular and luxurious oils that I just couldn't leave out of this book!

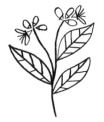

BENZOIN ABSOLUTE (*Styrax tonkinensis, Styrax benzoin*)
Source: Siam benzoin (*Styrax tonkinensis*) is preferred from Laos, Vietnam, Cambodia, China, Thailand; Sumatra benzoin (*Styrax benzoin*) is also from Sumatra, Java, and Malaysia
Distilled from: Gum resin, extracted with ethyl alcohol
Attributes: An amber oil, very thick and sticky, with a soft, sweet, vanilla perfumelike scent. It can be used as a base note to prolong the aroma of a personal scent (because it's not as costly as vanilla or amber).
Safety: It's gentle on skin when diluted, but it's not recommended for menopausal women.
Recommendations: *With its warming, decongesting, antiseptic, diuretic, and astringent properties,* this oil can be used if you need more help getting over a cough—along with pine, spruce, or fir—since it works as an effective expectorant. It is also a great oil to put in your all-over, everyday body oil (along with another astringent oil, like cypress) because it helps reduce fluid buildup in the legs and abdomen—a side effect of sitting for long periods. Also, take it with you when you travel and use it in your personal perfume inventions—it's a classic.

BERGAMOT (*Citrus aurantium* var. *bergamia*)
Source: Italy, Mediterranean region
Cold-pressed from: Peels of the unripe fruit
Attributes: A thin, light green oil known for its inclusion in Earl Grey tea, and has a cheerful citrusy scent on its own. It can be used as a top note for a natural room fragrance or in a fresh, personal scent applied to clothes.

Safety: The bergapten in this oil is highly photosensitizing, even twenty-four hours after application: it causes sunburn if you wear it in the sun. Dilute it with other essential oils and fatty oils. You can also purchase bergapten-free bergamot to avoid sun damage.

Recommendations: *With its cooling, relaxing, sedating, antidepressant, and antianxiety properties,* this oil is used as an inhalant to lift mood or control appetite, in baths to prepare for worry-free sleep, and in diffusers to bring a sense of well-being into the room. As an antiviral, it combines with ravensara for an effective cold sore relief, or with tea tree and lavender for shingles. This is a happy oil that puts almost everyone at ease and was grown in every medieval garden.

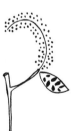

BIRCH, SWEET (*Betula lenta*)

Source: New England and northern Georgia in the United States, Canada (Don't use what comes from Europe or China—these are different, endangered varieties.)

Distilled from: Inner bark

Attributes: A sharp, strong oil that smells like root beer.

Safety: It can irritate the skin; use only a small amount in a blend with other essential oils and dilute in fatty oils. Avoid prolonged use; it may interact with some medications. It is not for use by anyone with a kidney condition; during pregnancy, childbirth, or lactation; or on children up to age five.

Recommendations: *With its warming, powerful analgesic, diuretic, and circulatory-stimulating properties,* this oil is an ideal choice for muscle spasms, injuries, chronic pain, and arthritis (though use peppermint instead if the joints are hot, red, or inflamed). Use it in your travel blend or sports blend—think of it as an ACE bandage with a topical pain reliever for injuries.

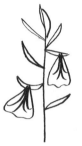

CARDAMOM (*Elettaria cardamomum*)
Source: India, Sri Lanka
Distilled from: Seeds
Attributes: A pale yellow to clear, watery oil with a spicy scent we associate with Indian cooking and exotic, woodsy perfumes. It works as a middle note for a personal scent.
Safety: Dilute in fatty oils. Avoid using it during menopause—it's too hot. *Not* for use around infants.
Recommendations: *With its warming, decongesting, muscle-relaxing, digestive, and soothing yet brain-stimulating properties,* this grounding oil is used to ease coughs, alleviate reflux, and quell nausea. If you use it as a personal or room deodorant, you can lift your mind out of a fog and improve your concentration. For a healthier gut, an organic drop can be used as an occasional substitute for ginger in juices, smoothies, or added to vegan baked goods.

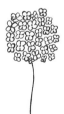

CARROT (*Daucus carota*)
Source: France, India, Egypt
Distilled from: Seeds
Attributes: An amber orange oil with a strong, earthy scent that needs to be combined with flower essential oils to make it pleasant to use.

Safety: Avoid during pregnancy and lactation.

Recommendations: *With its cooling, hepatic-stimulating, diuretic, and purifying properties,* this oil is for the skin and the liver. In a face oil, it reduces puffiness and, with its loads of provitamin A, regenerates and soothes sunburned, mature, and sensitive skin. Dilute it as a massage oil for a depleted liver, brittle nails, poor vision, and dizziness. The beauty that comes from this grounding oil will radiate from your contented mind.

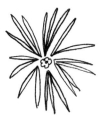

CEDARWOOD, ATLAS (*Cedrus atlantica*)

Source: Morocco (in ancient times, Lebanon cedars)

Distilled from: Wood chips and sawdust

Attributes: A pale yellow oil with a spicy, woodsy, soft scent that has more complexity than a cedar closet odor. Use it as base note to add gentle richness to wood, needle, and spice oils in a personal scent.

Safety: Avoid during pregnancy or lactation.

Recommendations: *With its cooling, antiseptic, antifungal, decongesting, and diuretic properties,* this oil is more than just an insect repellent for your closet. Use it when you're getting over a cough, in your neti pot during a cleanse, and in your shampoo or skin-brushing sequence to bring your life back into focus. It also gives a grounding effect to your travel kit basics, whether you anoint it in the center of your chest before bed or in your morning shower. Substitute: Moroccan *Cedrus atlantica,* Himalayan *Cedrus deodara,* and Virginian *Juniperus virginiana,* but they are not quite the same in their therapeutic benefits.

CHAMOMILE, German (blue) (*Matricaria recutita*) and Roman (*Anthemis nobilis*)

Source: France, Spain, Morocco, Egypt, Bavaria for the German variety

Distilled from: Flowers with stems

Attributes: German chamomile is dark blue-green and viscous with a strongly herbaceous, earthy scent. Roman chamomile is amber with a sweet, herbaceous scent that works well with other flower essential oils.

Safety: Avoid this oil if you are allergic to chamomile or ragweed.

Recommendations: *With its cooling and superior anti-inflammatory, antihistamine, and relaxing properties,* German chamomile is used for allergies; on inflamed areas caused by burns or allergies, like itchy, puffy eyes; and on inflamed, painful, arthritic joints, especially when symptoms are worse at night (like with TMJ). *With its appealing scent and gentleness,* Roman chamomile is the one for your daily face oil. It is a nurturing and calming oil to use during pregnancy, especially if you are having a hard time easing out of your hectic schedule to prepare for the baby. Both chamomile oils soothe skin when it's under stress. Substitute: Cape chamomile (*Eriocephalus punctulatus*) as an alternative to German (blue) chamomile.

CLARY SAGE (*Salvia sclarea*)

Source: France, Morocco, England

Distilled from: Flowering tops and leaves

Attributes: A clear, watery oil that is very sweet, musky, and herbaceous. Use it as a middle note in a personal scent; you may prefer it blended rather than all by itself.

Safety: It's not for use during pregnancy. Avoid it when drinking alcohol, because it will increase drunkenness before you know it.

Recommendations: *With its cooling, lavenderlike, antianxiety, and sedating properties and its euphoric, hormone-balancing effect,* it is an important sleep enhancer and stress reducer, affecting the dopamine levels in the brain and lowering blood pressure. When hormonal swings cause emotions to run high or mood to sink low, couple this oil with geranium or ylang-ylang for use during slow breathing inhalations and you will feel better. It also works wonders on wrinkles and acne, and it is a lovely deodorant.

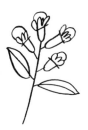

CLOVE (*Syzygium aromaticum*)

Source: Madagascar, Tanzania

Distilled from: Dried flowers, buds, and leaves

Attributes: A clear to yellow, watery oil that smells like the cloves used in cooking but stronger! Add it as a middle note to heat up a personal scent (see the following safety dilution ratio).

Safety: It can irritate or burn the skin or gums. Always dilute it to less than 1% in a fatty oil, or dilute it in other essential oils and then dilute the blend in jojoba oil at a ratio of one to four. It is not for long-term use and not for use during pregnancy, childbirth, or lactation, or on young children or menopausal women.

Recommendations: *With its hot, very powerful, antiviral, antifungal, and pain-relieving properties,* this oil has been used traditionally for oral hygiene and numbing pain relief (dilute it in coconut oil for a mouthwash and baking soda for a toothpaste). Use it at the first sign of a gum or tooth infection and in workout shoes to prevent athlete's foot. To build more resilience, add a drop of clove to a blend of grapefruit and bay laurel and put a drop of the blend on your shower floor for your morning ritual or put it in your goblet at work.

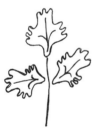

CORIANDER (*Coriandrum sativum*)
Source: Spain, Ukraine, Hungary, Russia
Distilled from: Seeds
Attributes: A clear, watery oil with an elegant, spicy middle note for your body care products and as an enlivening personal scent.
Safety: Slightly photosensitizing: it causes sunburn if you wear it in the sun.
Recommendations: *With its pain-relieving, decongesting, antibacterial, and digestive properties,* this oil is useful to inhale while recovering from an intestinal bug, food poisoning, or an eating disorder. Add it to your pain-relieving blend if you tend to get fluid in your joints or worry about weight gain when

you take time off from your workout to heal an injury. On the bright side, it is a beautiful sleep, mood, concentration, and libido enhancer!

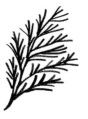

CYPRESS (*Cupressus sempervirens*)
Source: France, Italy, North Africa, Spain, Portugal
Distilled from: Needles, twigs, and cones
Attributes: A clear, watery oil and a spicy middle note that smells better than pine.
Safety: May cause skin irritation if stored in direct light or heat for over two years.
Recommendations: *With its slightly cooling astringent, diuretic, and vasoconstricting properties,* this oil can be used for cellulite and "draining dampness," a Traditional Chinese Medicine term for those who tend to retain water, sweat easily, have digestive issues, have chronic congestion, or injure easily due to overly loose joints, often caused by eating too many sweet foods and a lack of exercise. As the first step in getting back to exercise, use it in an all-over body oil with a walking meditation and do lots of slow breathing inhalations in the shower. If you start coughing, visualize your lungs clearing out as you let go of the past.

EUCALYPTUS (*Eucalyptus globulus, Eucalyptus radiata, eucalyptus citriodora*)
Source: Australia, Portugal, Spain, France; *Eucalyptus radiata* is also from China, India. Citriodora also from Madagascar.

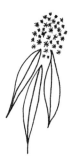

Distilled from: Leaves and twigs

Attributes: A clear, watery oil with an unmistakable spicy, camphorlike, very strong aroma.

Safety: It's not for use during lactation or where babies could inhale the oil or on children under the age of five. Combine with other oils and/or dilute.

Recommendations: *With its antiviral, antibacterial, decongesting punch and its anti-inflammatory and pain-relieving properties,* this oil is a staple for cold and flu season. Inhale it up to five times a day. Dilute it as a treatment oil and apply it to the shoulders for aches and pains. *Eucalyptus radiata* is for earaches (dripped on a cotton ball), sinus congestion, sore throats, and swollen glands—where a cold or the flu often takes hold. As your breathing passages clear, stamina returns and the impossible seems doable once again. In summer, use insect-repelling lemon eucalyptus (citriodora) instead.

FIR, *see* Pine

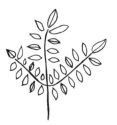

FRANKINCENSE (*Boswellia carteri*)

Source: Lebanon, Africa, Iran, Arabian Peninsula

Distilled from: Milky white oleoresin found in the trunk of the plant

Attributes: A clear to yellow-brown, watery to viscous oil with a spicy, earthy scent. It can be a balsamic base note that will make a personal scent last longer.

Safety: Safe for all purposes.

Recommendations: This supreme meditation oil has

pain-relieving, skin-healing, expectorant, anti-infectious, and sedating properties that prepare the mind for peaceful and tranquil thoughts—and sleep—by calming nerves, anxiety, irritability, and mental chatter. It relieves coughs, sinus infections, and chest tightness for deeper breathing; is known for its ability to heal wounds and scars, both physical and emotional; and soothes depression. With five thousand years as the basis for spiritual abundance, this oil can't be ignored.

GERANIUM (*Pelargonium graveolens*)
Source: Réunion Island, Morocco, North Africa
Distilled from: Leaves
Attributes: A clear to light greenish-yellow oil with a very strong, rose-sweet scent. A small amount works as a middle note with other oils for a personal scent.
Safety: Safe for all purposes. Possible interaction with diabetes medication.
Recommendations: *With its antifungal, anti-inflammatory, immunostimulant, detoxifying, and antianxiety properties,* this calming de-stressor is an extremely versatile oil. Dilute it for use in skin care and as a treatment oil for hypertension, varicose veins, athlete's foot, stretch marks, lymphatic congestion (caused by travel, lack of exercise, and excess tension that depletes the immune system), menopause, and PMS. Known to "knock at the heart's door," it welcomes you back into your rich emotional life after you've been stuck in your head too long. Try it at the end of the day to switch gears.

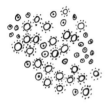

HELICHRYSUM (*Helichrysum angustifolium*), also known as immortelle or everlast
Source: Corsica, Bosnia, Herzegovina
Distilled from: Flowers
Attributes: A yellow to orange, watery oil with a pungent scent best balanced in a blend.
Safety: This oil is okay to use 1 drop topically undiluted, but I recommend diluting.
Recommendations: *With its renowned skin-regenerating, healing, anti-inflammatory, and pain-relieving properties,* this expensive oil has the best antiaging elements essential oils can provide. Stretch a 5-milliliter bottle to a pint size by combining it with three to five of your other favorite essential oils before adding the mixture to rosehip seed oil and jojoba oil (make a big batch and store it in the fridge). Or use it in a more concentrated form for scar reduction. For wound care, use it right on the injury. Make a pain-relieving blend with peppermint, or mix it with a few drops of German chamomile to keep on hand for any and all sprains, strains, spasms, and injuries. Just like first aid in a bottle, use this oil first and watch it work miracles!

HYSSOP DECUMBENS (*Hyssopus officinalis* var. *decumbens*)
Source: Hungary, France
Distilled from: Flowering tops and leaves
Attributes: A clear, watery oil with a spicy, sweet,

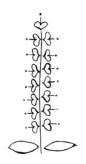

camphorlike top note that blends well with lavender, geranium, and/or citrus in a home deodorizer.

Safety: Safe for all uses unless you confuse this oil with the toxic variation: hyssop *officinalis*, which is neurotoxic.

Recommendations: *With its cooling and very powerful antiviral properties,* this oil decongests the lungs and is commonly used to alleviate allergies, coughs, and bronchitis. It is distinctly detoxifying and cleansing because it is eliminated through the lungs instead of through the skin; make sure to diffuse it. Use this oil as the breathable, premier purifier in lieu of burning sage.

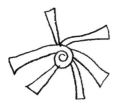

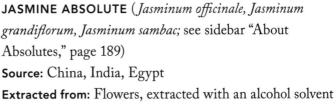

JASMINE ABSOLUTE (*Jasminum officinale, Jasminum grandiflorum, Jasminum sambac;* see sidebar "About Absolutes," page 189)

Source: China, India, Egypt

Extracted from: Flowers, extracted with an alcohol solvent

Attributes: A brown and extremely thick oil, it makes a pungent, sweet base note to a personal scent.

Safety: Although this oil is safe for all uses, it is often an adulterated oil, which can cause an adverse reaction. Source organic only and expect to pay more—it's worth it.

Recommendations: *With its superior antidepressant, aphrodisiac, and narcotic effects,* jasmine will safely intoxicate you and everyone around you. It's too intense to use by itself; add flowers, citrus, or spices to *Jasminum grandiflorum,* especially for a beautiful body care blend. Although it is tempting to use this oil nonstop, use *Jasminum sambac* (night-blooming jasmine) only when you need it most, like when you're getting back in the groove after being sick or when you're exhausted from too much travel or anxiety. During childbirth, use jasmine when the labor has been prolonged, and then later inhale during the breast-feeding phase.

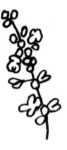

LAVENDER (*Lavandula angustifolia*)

Source: Provence region of France, Bulgaria (Always buy the best lavender and only substitute with the lavandin variation if nothing else is available.)

Distilled from: Flowering tops, picked at night or in the early morning

Attributes: A clear, watery oil with an herbaceous, sweet middle to top note for a personal scent.

Safety: Safe for all uses, though not for use on a wound that is still bleeding.

Recommendations: *With its anti-infectious, antiviral, antifungal, pain-relieving, muscle-relaxing, and mood- and sleep-enhancing properties,* this all-purpose oil is all you may need for a while. You can use it to treat respiratory infections, to heal wounds and burns, for pain relief, to calm your nerves, and to restore deep breathing. When you are feeling creative, lavender can make a new oil blend sing. Like milk in your coffee, it takes off the rough edges and harmonizes disparate scents. However, some people absolutely don't like it! For the rest of us, including kids and pregnant women, when it is diffused, it gives us the feeling of a clean, clear space to think and be well.

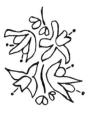

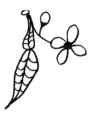

LEMON (*Citrus limon*), **lime** (*Citrus aurantifolia*), **grapefruit** (*Citrus × paradisi*)

Source: Italy, United States, West Indies

Cold-pressed from: Peels—use organic only!

Attributes: The lemon oil is clear to yellow; the lime, clear; and the grapefruit, clear to pink with pink grapefruit as its scent.

Safety: All of these oils are photosensitizing. Stay out of the sun for twelve hours after applying to avoid sunburn. Store in the refrigerator to avoid oxidation and possible skin irritation. Grapefruit is the gentlest oil on the skin.

Recommendations: *With their cooling, antiseptic, antidepressant, diuretic, and antioxidant-loaded properties,* these citrus oils stimulate and give you a fresh feeling. They are perfect for every day. Pick the one you love and definitely inhale and diffuse it to gently cleanse your liver and knock out those free radicals. A dieter's best friends, lemon regulates blood sugar and grapefruit helps metabolize fats. You can safely ingest these oils simply by eating the rind of the organic fruits. Dilute them as per a body oil to treat cellulite or avoid fluid retention when traveling. To keep your home or workspace feeling clean and cheerful, you can't go wrong with any combination of these oils plus some hyssop decumbens, bergamot, or lavender.

LITSEA CUBEBA (*Litsea cubeba*), also known as may chang

Source: China

Distilled from: Fruit

Attributes: A yellow oil that smells like, but should not be

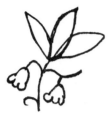

confused with, lemon balm. It can be a very strong middle note and requires a lot of top to dilute it in a personal scent.

Safety: This oil can irritate the skin; dilute it with other essential oils and fatty oils. It is not for use during pregnancy or lactation, or on young children and may interact with some medications.

Recommendations: *With its analgesic and anti-inflammatory properties,* this important oil works in all pain preparations to warm the muscles, reduce swelling, and relieve pain—especially for lower back issues. It is used in Traditional Chinese Medicine to help the body adjust to changes in temperature and climate as well as motion sickness, making this an excellent oil for travel.

MANDARIN, *see* Orange

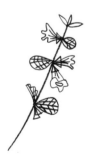

MELISSA (*Melissa officinalis*), also known as lemon balm

Source: France, Germany (Buy organic only; this oil is often adulterated.)

Distilled from: Leaves—produces an excellent hydrosol

Attributes: A yellow, watery oil that is a sweet, lemony, herbaceous middle note.

Safety: Always dilute in a fatty oil and store in the refrigerator. Like needle oils, it can irritate skin if it is old or improperly stored. It's not for use during pregnancy or lactation, or on young children.

Recommendations: *With its relaxing, sedating, and powerful antiviral properties,* this expensive oil is worth it when used to dispel a period of extreme anxiety and stress—the kind that erodes composure, reason, and trust, making sleep unattainable and blood pressure rise, even affecting digestion and fertility (use the oil *before* trying to get pregnant). Use melissa twice a day in a very diluted body oil along with a hydrosol for instant soothing. Inhale the undiluted oil to aid sleep or relieve migraines. Have faith in its healing properties; the sixteenth-century Swiss-German physician Paracelsus called it the "elixir of life."

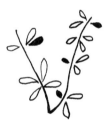

MYRRH (*Commiphora myrrha*)
Source: Somalia, Oman, Libya
Distilled from: Gum resin
Attributes: A yellow to dark brown, very thick, sticky paste (it may need to be warmed before use). It adds a bitter, spicy, earthy base note to personal blends that makes the scent last.
Safety: Safe for all purposes. Not for use during pregnancy and lactation.
Recommendations: *With its cooling, antifungal, antiviral, and anti-inflammatory properties,* it's commonly used, along with clove, for oral hygiene in toothpaste and also for foot care and hygiene. Another ancient oil that was used for coughs, myrrh can be used today with lemon eucalyptus for a summer flu. It was classically combined with frankincense for meditation practice, as the way to begin the process of relaxing the body and tuning out external distractions, making it another useful oil for anxiety and mental focus.

NIAOULI, *see* Tea Tree

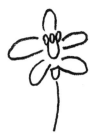

NEROLI (*Citrus aurantium* var. *amara*)
Source: France, Morocco, Egypt, Italy
Distilled from: Flowers of the bitter orange tree (the peels of the fruit and leaves of the tree produce bitter orange and petitgrain essential oils)
Attributes: A pale yellow oil with a sweet, floral-citrus aroma that entices many but not all. It is both a joyous and grounding base note for a very personal scent—a true luxury oil with a price that matches.
Safety: It's safe for all purposes, but it's not for exclusive long-term use since it can lower energy levels. If you wish to use it in an everyday personal scent, alternate it with jasmine, rose, or coriander.
Recommendations: *With its cooling, calming, and regenerative properties,* this oil, when used for skin care, won't irritate even the most sensitive skin. It is an ideal base for mature, sensitive, and combination skin, and for treating rosacea and wrinkles. There are cheaper ways to heal scars and stretch marks, but indulge in it if you can, since this oil will lift you out of your depression and help you sleep beautifully. For an elegant pick-me-up, put a drop on your sternum and feel your chest open and lift for better posture.

ORANGE, sweet, blood, or bitter (*Citrus sinensis*, bitter is *Citrus aurantium* var. *amara*), **mandarin** (*Citrus nobilis*)

Source: Italy, France, Florida, Mediterranean region

Cold-pressed from: Peels of the fruits

Attributes: Orange, watery oils that smell just like their fruits. They can be a top note for a personal scent that everyone will love.

Safety: To avoid skin sensitizing, store in the refrigerator like other citrus oils. It's an affordable oil everyone loves, though not for exclusive long-term use since it can lower energy levels.

Recommendations: *With their digestive, sedative, and antidepressant properties,* these oils are nature's way of counteracting depression, uplifting your mood without overstimulating. Sleep is time for the body to rest and digest, making these oils ideal in a blend used before bed, whether inhaled for sleep (sweet) or applied during an abdominal massage (bitter). Mandarin is the best on the skin and often appeals to children. Tangerine (*Citrus Reticulata*) is often used instead of mandarin, and both stimulate digestion, though the more pungent bitter orange is the most stimulating.

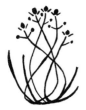

PALMAROSA (*Cymbopogon martinii*)

Source: Madagascar, Brazil, Nepal, India

Distilled from: Grass

Attributes: A clear, watery oil with a gentle, rosy scent. It's a top note that can dilute a strong oil in a personal scent.

Safety: Safe for all purposes. Store in the refrigerator to avoid oxidation and possible skin irritation.

Recommendations: *With its very cooling, antibacterial, anti-inflammatory, and cellular-regenerative properties,* this oil is frequently used in skin preparations to reduce redness (rosacea), dryness, and even inflamed patches due to dermatitis, eczema, or psoriasis, and it is gentle enough for mild topical infections. It is also used in massage blends where there is nerve pain with excess tension, as with sciatica and chronic jaw clenching, or with teeth grinding that causes inflammation in the temporomandibular joint, which radiates nerve pain to the face, neck, eyes, and head, even causing dizziness. Diffuse or drop the oil on the back of your neck (with peppermint) for jet lag and to cool down after travel.

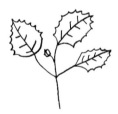

PATCHOULI (*Pogostemon cablin;* also known as *Pogostemon patchouli*)
Source: Indonesia, India, Burma (Myanmar), Brazil
Distilled from: Dried, fermented leaves
Attributes: A dark amber oil with an herbaceous, familiar scent that is extremely mutable—it is different with each distiller and changes with age. For a warm, earthy, musky (but not animal) base note in a personal blend, use only the tiniest amount.
Safety: It's safe for all purposes but a possible anti-coagulant and interaction with blood thinners.
Recommendations: *With its many therapeutic properties, including its use as an immunity and digestive aid,* patchouli, you would think, would be a great everything oil. Stop! This oil is so highly concentrated you need only a drop in a

blend, making it perfect for skin care. Use it for mature, dry, cracked, or sweaty skin, especially in the summer months (see also "Cypress," page 197). Add it to macadamia or olive oil for elderly skin care. But this oil truly excels at steadfastly elevating your mood as it enhances your sensuality, sexuality, and fertility (perhaps this is why it has been commonly paired with cannabis oil!).

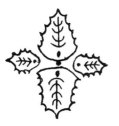

PEPPERMINT (*Mentha × piperita*)
Source: France, Italy (Get the best you can afford.)
Distilled from: Leaves
Attributes: A clear oil with a distinctive, strong menthol scent that ranges from a candy smell (the cheap oils) to a complex, herbaceous top note.
Safety: Avoid this oil during childbirth and lactation, and keep it away from children under five. Test it for sensitivity if you are using it undiluted. It is not for use on the face, and it can cause acid reflux if ingested.
Recommendations: *With its opposing actions—cooling and warming, calming and stimulating, and relaxing and inspiring—*this oil does what only nature can do. This highly adaptogenic oil can relieve mental fatigue and prepare you for sleep, open your sinuses and reduce fever, and alleviate bloating and nausea. It repels insects and eases itching. It is also the antidote to long hours at the computer or standing all day—and loved by performers because it energizes while it helps combat stage fright. If you are tired of your lavender fix-all, switch to peppermint. It's like airing out your brain to create space for new ideas.

PETITGRAIN (*Citrus aurantium* var. *amara*)
Source: Italy, France, Madagascar
Distilled from: Leaves and stems of the bitter orange tree
Attributes: A clear, watery oil used as a top note in French perfumery since the seventeenth century. Explore blending it with some of your favorite oils.
Safety: Safe for all purposes.
Recommendations: *With its antidepressant, calming, and relaxing properties,* this oil should be in any antidepressant or antianxiety blend because you can use it long-term (unlike the oranges). It also works to strengthen memory. Apply it undiluted with peppermint to the center of your chest at the beginning of your day and/or with a flower essential oil at the end of your day and notice your mood evening out. For skin care, put a drop on a cotton ball, then dip the ball into water for an instant toner to tighten the pores.

PINE (*Pinus sylvestris*), **black spruce** (*Picea mariana*), **fir** (*Abies alba*)
Source: Europe
Distilled from: Needles and cones
Attributes: All three are clear, watery oils. Pine smells like itself; spruce is softer and earthy; fir is the beauty in the bunch: a spicy, sweet middle note for a personal scent, and it is especially helpful to use it while grieving or getting over a loss.

Safety: These are safe for all purposes unless the oil is more than two years old (it can irritate the skin). I recommend diluting.

Recommendations: *With their decongesting properties,* these grounding oils are used in bath and massage oils for anti-inflammatory and pain-relieving effects, and in chest rubs for coughs, asthma, and allergies. I always add fir to brighten the blend. But when you are burned out (your adrenals are depleted) or a cold has turned into a respiratory infection, get the major lift needed from the antibacterial, hormone-boosting punch of pine and/or spruce.

RAVENSARA (*Ravensara aromatica*)

Source: Madagascar

Distilled from: Leaves

Attributes: A clear, watery oil with a eucalyptuslike scent.

Safety: It's safe for all purposes.

Recommendations: *With its decongesting and powerful antiviral properties,* this oil should go into all your summer and winter remedies because it works with head colds and chest colds at once, not to mention the aches and pains that accompany these bugs. Known for its effectiveness on herpes and shingles, this oil is worth a try since antibiotics can't help you with viral infections, and you can diffuse it as well. Not to be confused with ravintsara (*cinnamomum camphora*, also called ho leaf oil).

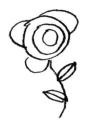

ROSE (*Rosa × damascena, Rosa × centifolia*)
Source: Bulgaria (the best source), Morocco, and Turkey for *Rosa × damascena* (known as rose otto); Provence for the absolute *Rosa × centifolia*. (Be skeptical of bargain brands from other sources since they are often adulterated.)
Distilled from: Flowers
Attributes: A clear to pale yellow oil that is waxy and thick.
Safety: It is gentle, though do not use it on your face if you have rosacea, and always dilute the absolute.
Recommendations: *With its liver-supportive, antidepressant, and soothing properties,* this oil is supreme for the heart and your emotional wellness. Dilute it in jojoba oil and put a drop in the center of your chest when you need a hug, are pregnant (second or third trimester only), or are preparing for sleep. Dilute it more with rosehip seed oil and use it in skin care mixtures for its glowing results. Use it in loving meditation to help you stop judging yourself and cultivate trust that everything is just as it was meant to be.

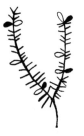

ROSEMARY (*Rosmarinus officinalis*)
Source: Italy, other Mediterranean and Adriatic countries
Distilled from: Leaves and flowering tops
Attributes: A clear, watery oil with a spicy, camphorlike scent you know from the plant.
Safety: Avoid if you have high blood pressure. Use in small amounts. Not for use during pregnancy or lactation, or around anyone with epilepsy or young children where they could inhale the oil.

Recommendations: *With its warming, decongesting, stimulating, and toning effect on the liver, heart, lung, and blood circulation,* this reanimating oil is frequently used for mental focus; hair care; care of the hands and feet; treatment of cellulite, flu, and colds; and general treatment of a "damp" personality (see "Cypress," page 197). There are a few types of rosemary: verbenone is the one for skin care; cineole is the one for respiratory issues. However, this enthusiastic oil isn't for everyone, like workaholics and people who are high-strung, because it is very stimulating. (It's not a Gillerman family oil!) Such people would be better off with eucalyptus, peppermint, and/or pine or spruce.

SANDALWOOD (*santalum spicatum A., santalum austrocaledonicum Vieill*)
Source: Australia (*spicatum A.*), most similar to Indian endangered oil from Mysore (*Santalum album*), New Caledonia and New Zealand (*austrocaledonicum*), Hawaii (*paniculatum*)
Distilled from: Wood and roots
Attributes: A clear to pale yellow, thick, viscous oil with a very mild woodsy scent that is a base note for a soft-smelling personal scent.
Safety: Safe for all purposes.
Recommendations: *With its emollient, diuretic, and relaxing effects,* this oil takes the tension out of your facial expressions, reduces puffiness, and soothes the skin after sunburn. When inhaled, it softly eases into the lungs to deepen and relax your breath. Historically, it was used in meditation by anointing it on the chest after myrrh had been diffused, to bring quiet

to the mind, making it a great sleep and antianxiety oil. The kind of renewed vitality this peaceful oil can bring is so luxurious, sensual, and grounding, it gives you more time to enjoy the moment.

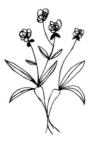

SPIKENARD (*Nardostachys jatamansi*)
Source: Himalayas, India
Distilled from: Rhizomes (stems that live predominantly underground, like ginger)
Attributes: A dark amber, thick oil with a woodsy, musky, heavy scent that takes a bit of getting used to but is worth it. I dilute it with lavender.
Safety: Safe for all purposes.
Recommendations: *With its significant sedating and relaxing effect,* this oil is for deep sleep, especially when noise, travel, and overtiredness factor into extreme wakefulness. And it is a much easier oil to find, can be used long-term, and is less costly than valerian. It works simultaneously by calming anxiety and cooling emotions that would otherwise keep your mind racing. For insomnia associated with menopause, it is recommended with clary sage. It is also used in religious practices to help people surrender and relax.

SPRUCE, *see* Pine

TEA TREE (*Melaleuca alternifolia*), **niaouli** (*Melaleuca quinquenervia, Melaleuca viridiflora,* or MQV)
Source: Australia, New Zealand, New Caledonia

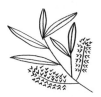

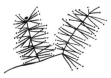

Distilled from: Leaves

Attributes: Both oils are clear and watery. Tea tree has a very strong, distinct, eucalyptuslike, masculine scent. Niaouli has a sweeter, eucalyptuslike scent.

Safety: Tea tree is a safe, gentle oil when used diluted. Avoid using niaouli on or near children and infants to prevent inhalation, but for adults it is safe for all purposes.

Recommendations: *With their cooling and well-researched disinfecting, anti-viral properties,* these widely available melaleuca oils are your go-to for immune support and treatment of infections in the mouth or on the feet, wounds, a sore throat, and ailments of the chest. Choose one of them to take with you when traveling to sanitize your plane seat or hotel shower. Milder tea tree is an antifungal commonly used for thrush or candida, and it is safe for use during pregnancy and on children over one year old (see Dilution Chart, page 46). Niaouli is the one for allergies and PMS, and for use on teenagers especially for acne-prone skin. If you feel like you are always getting sick and just can't get healthy, add one of these oils in a dilution and use it in your daily self-care routine. (Other types of melaleuca oils include harsher cajeput. Gentler rosalina and variations of niaouli have limited availability.)

VANILLA ABSOLUTE (*Vanilla planifolia*) (see sidebar "About Absolutes," page 189)

Source: Madagascar

Distilled from: Resin (The CO_2 extracted oil has an aroma closer to the scent of the familiar cooking extract. I prefer

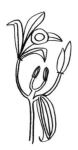

the sweet-smelling vanilla absolute, extracted with ethyl alcohol.)

Attributes: An amber oil with a warm, soft, sweet scent that's a little different from the synthetic vanilla you're used to in perfumes and body care products. It works perfectly as a base note in a personal scent. To save on cost, you can use benzoin instead, but that oil has different therapeutic effects.

Safety: Safe for all purposes.

Recommendations: *With its emotionally cathartic properties,* this oil is needed in our lives and in our personal care products to remind us to let go, to feel more emotionally connected to our loved ones, and to feel more socially at ease. I used it to help my dog let go and pass all on her own. Experiment freely!

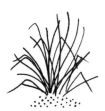

VETIVER (*Vetiveria zizanioides*)

Source: El Salvador, Haiti, Sri Lanka

Distilled from: Dried roots

Attributes: A dark red-brown oil that is thicker than molasses. It works as a base note in a personal scent and prolongs the aroma on your body for two days, always changing slightly. Dilute it with lavender and other oils before blending it with a fatty oil.

Safety: Safe for all purposes; always use diluted.

Recommendations: *With its muscle-relaxing and calming properties,* this multifunctional oil strengthens the immune system while it reduces anxieties. It's an effective massage oil because it stimulates blood circulation (I have even used it to prevent frostbite in New England), relaxes joints, and helps heal injuries. Remember the discussion of essential oils affecting the limbic system? This oil goes there to release fear as it releases you from genetically programmed tension patterns at the root of your pain and stress.

YLANG-YLANG (*Cananga odorata*), always choose ylang-ylang extra or ylang-ylang complete
Source: Madagascar, Indonesia, Comoros, Réunion Island
Distilled from: Flowers
Attributes: A clear, watery oil with a very strong and sweet vanillalike floral top that works as a middle or base note in a personal scent. Do not use it by itself.
Safety: It's gentle, but always use it in very small amounts in combination with other oils to avoid skin irritation or a reaction to its sweet scent. I don't recommend it if you have extremely low blood pressure or you are constantly cold.
Recommendations: *With its well-known aphrodisiac and anti-depressant yet soothing and relaxing properties,* this oil can bring joy—so long as you dilute it with other essential oils! It lowers blood pressure, calms heart palpitations, soothes anxiety, and even helps you dream more vividly, a modern wonder you can add to your shampoo, body wash, soap, or other skin care items (especially for treating acne). If you feel restless or agitated and find yourself withdrawing, take a bath or make a chest rub with this oil and get dressed for fun!

CONCLUSION

Essential oils are like the qi—the breath, or life—of a plant. Just as any plant does, we constantly need to adapt to our surroundings. Luckily, we're able to partner with plants to help us. If you can imagine how strong our connection to plants can be, since we live together on this earth, you just might find out that the use of essential oils is even more important today than it has been in centuries past.

So many people I have met and worked with have changed their lives as a result of using essential oils. Hundreds of people tell me they sleep better, worry less, breathe deeper, smile more, have less pain, stand up taller, have radiant skin, and have developed a greater appreciation of their sense of smell. Each time, I listen to their stories and hear their gratitude. Our silent plant partners have a loud voice if we're willing to listen. Aromatic healing offers strong results, with a peaceful resolve. Then I feel myself stepping back and saying, "See what essential oils can do?"

Now I step back for you, so you can have your own experience.

Be well and enjoy your oils.

Peace and love,

Hope

ACKNOWLEDGMENTS

I have so enjoyed every moment of this collaboration with HarperElixir's team of perfectionists and especially with senior editor Libby Edelson, who welcomed me with her true warmth and brilliance right from the start, and for all that she has freely given to this book. I'd also like to thank Claudia Boutote, Melinda Mullen, Adia Colar, Amy VanLangen, Suzanne Quist, and Anissa Elmerraji. Incredible gratitude to Meghan Stevenson for offering her revisions and guidance with honesty and support. To my dedicated and wise agent, Katherine Latshaw at Folio, and to Michael Sterling and Katherine for helping to make this book happen! To medievalist Dorothy Gillerman, who reads Dioscorides and knows the truth about Mary Magdalene. Thanks to Aimee Majoros, Simone Federman, and Eugenia Semjonova for your moving stories, and again to Simone, John E., Mary Ann, and Ellen, who have heard it all so many times—thank you, thank you, thank you. Finally, to Alison Oliver for lending her humor, her nature-loving spirit, and her endless artistry to this book.

RESOURCES

SITES TO EXPLORE FOR PURCHASING THE HIGHEST-QUALITY, SINGLE ORGANIC, AND WILD-CRAFTED AND SYNERGISTIC BLENDS ONLINE:

• Original Swiss Aromatics for organic single oils and some fatty oils, hydrosols, and synergistic blends from the work of biochemist Kurt Schnaubelt. Associated with the Pacific Institute of Aromatherapy. www.originalswissaromatics.com

• Eden Botanicals. Buy single oils only—they have a great sampling option and many absolutes for making your personal perfumes. www.edenbotanicals.com

• Organic Infusions for a large collection of organic hydrosols and fatty oils. www.organicinfusionswholesale.com

• The Lebermuth Company. They are primarily a wholesale fragrance company, but they carry quite a few organic essential oils and test their products thoroughly. They always welcome a phone call from an interested consumer looking to get a hold of the latest batch of lavender. Buy organic single oils only. www.lebermuth.com/store/

• National Association for Holistic Aromatherapy. Go to their marketplace for a list of aromatherapy businesses owned by trained aromatherapists. www.naha.org (Go to the Resources link under "Explore Aromatherapy.")

The better brands found in health food stores are Veriditas Botanicals and Simplers Botanicals. For store locations, see veriditasbotanicals.com and simplers.com.

WHERE TO BUY 5-MILLILITER AND 15-MILLILITER EUROPEAN DROPPERS AND 1-, 2-, AND 4-OUNCE BOSTON ROUNDS:

• E.D. Luce Packaging allows you to buy the quantity you want, though you will be buying the caps separately, so take your time on the site. Buy only dark-colored glass bottles and stay away from plastic bottles. www.essentialsupplies.com

HOW AND WHERE TO BUY YOUR BOTANICAL BEAUTY PRODUCTS, LIKE CLEANSING GELS, READY-MADE FACE OIL, MASKS, AND SCRUBS (LISTED ALPHABETICALLY):

- Credo Beauty
- The Detox Market
- Follain
- Green Line Beauty
- Spirit Beauty Lounge

Go into their stores, or get on the phone before you order, to get the benefit of their experienced and knowledgeable staff. Colloidal oatmeal can be ordered through products like Aveeno Active Naturals Soothing Bath Treatment; select fragrance free only (Note: Their other products are not as pure). It is a pure powder you can use well on your face.

FOR MORE ON GREEN MAKEUP:

- Go to Katey Denno's site, The Beauty of It Is . . . . www.thebeautyofitis.com
- Here is her list of no-nos I promised you:

Albumin	Phthalates
Bentonite	Propylene glycol
Butylated hydroxyanisole (BHA)	PVP/VA copolymer
and butylated hydroxytoluene (BHT)	Quaternium-15
Diazolidinyl urea	Sodium lauryl sulfate and
Dibutyl phthalate	sodium laureth sulfate
DMDM hydantoin	Stearalkonium chloride
Ethanolamine, DEA, MEA, and TEA	Talc
FD&C color pigments	Triclosan
Glycerin	Toluene
Imidazolidinyl urea	
Isopropyl alcohol	**In products for kids:**
Mineral oil	2-bromo-2-nitropropane-1,3-diol
PEG	BHA
Petroleum/petrolatum	Boric acid and sodium borate

BIBLIOGRAPHY

Amrita Aromatherapy, http://www.amrita.net

"Amy Cuddy, Power Poser." Game Changers. *Time* video, 5:58. Accessed September 14, 2015. http://content.time.com/time/specials/packages/article/0,28804,2091589_2092033_2109441,00.html.

Arzi, A., L. Sela, A. Green, G. Givaty, Y. Dagan, and N. Sobel. "The Influence of Odorants on Respiratory Patterns in Sleep." *Chemical Senses* 35, no. 1 (2010): 31–40.

Atsumi, T., and K. Tonosaki. "Smelling Lavender and Rosemary Increases Free Radical Scavenging Activity and Decreases Cortisol Level in Saliva." *Psychiatry Research* 150, no. 1 (2007): 89–96.

Bagetta G., L. A. Morrone, L. Rombolà, D. Amantea, R. Russo, L. Berliocchi, S. Sakurada, T. Sakurada, D. Rotiroti, and M. T. Corasaniti. "Neuropharmacology of the Essential Oil of Bergamot." *Fitoterapia* 81, no. 6 (2010): 453–61.

Battaglia, Salvatore. *The Complete Guide to Aromatherapy.* 2nd ed. Sydney, Australia: Perfect Potion Press, 2003.

Bhasin, M. K., J. A. Dusek, B.-H. Chang, M. G. Joseph, J. W. Denninger, G. L. Fricchione, H. Benson, and T. A. Libermann. "Relaxation Response Induces Temporal Transcriptome Changes in Energy Metabolism, Insulin Secretion, and Inflammatory Pathways." *PLoS One* 8, no. 5 (2013): e62817.

Bozin, B., N. Mimica-Dukic, I. Samojlik, and E. Jovin. "Antimicrobial and Antioxidant Properties of Rosemary and Sage (*Rosmarinus Officinalis L.* and *Salvia Officinalis L., Lamiaceae*) Essential Oils." *Journal of Agricultural and Food Chemistry* 55, no. 19 (2007): 7879–85.

Carson, C. F., B. D. Cookson, H. D. Farrelly, and T. V. Riley. "Susceptibility of Methicillin-Resistant Staphylococcus Aureus to the Essential Oil Melaleuca Alternifolia." *Journal of Antimicrobial Chemotherapy* 35, no. 3 (1995): 421–24.

Cash, B. D., M. S. Epstein, and S. M. Shah. "A Novel Delivery System of Peppermint Oil Is an Effective Therapy for Irritable Bowel Syndrome Symptoms." *Digestive Diseases and Sciences* (August 29, 2015).

Chuang, K.-J., H.-W. Chen, I.-J. Liu, H.-C. Chuang, and L.-Y. Lin. "The Effect of Essential Oil on Heart Rate and Blood Pressure Among Solus por Aqua Workers." *European Journal of Preventive Cardiology* 21, no. 7 (2012): 823–28.

Duan, D., L. Chen, X. Yang, and S. Jiao. "Antidepressant-Like Effect of Essential Oil Isolated from Toona Ciliata Roem. Var. Yunnanensis." *Journal of Natural Medicine* 69, no. 2 (2015): 191–97.

Edwards-Jones, V., R. Buck, S. G. Shawcross, M. M. Dawson, and K. Dunn. "The Effect of Essential Oils on Methicillin-Resistant Staphylococcus Aureus Using a Dressing Model." *Burns: Journal of the International Society for Burn Injuries* 30, no. 8 (2004): 772–77.

Favre-Godal, Q., E. F. Queiroz, and J. L. Wolfender. "Latest Developments in Assessing Antifungal Activity Using TLC-Autobiography: A Review." *Journal of the Association of Official Analytical Chemists* 96, no. 6 (2013): 1175–88.

Gardulf, A., I. Wohlfart, and R. Gustafson. "A Prospective Cross-over Field Trial Shows Protection of Lemon Eucalyptus Extract Against Tick Bites." *Journal of Medical Entomology* 41, no. 6 (2004): 1064–67.

Hansraj, K. "Assessment of Stresses in the Cervical Spine Caused by Posture and Position of the Head," *Surgical Technology International* 25 (2014). "Amy Cuddy and associates showed that high-power posture posers experienced elevations in testosterone, increases in serotonin, decreases in cortisol, and increased feelings of power and tolerance for risk taking. Low-power posture posers exhibited the opposite pattern."

Hongratanaworakit, T. "Relaxing Effect of Rose Oil on Humans." *Natural Product Communications* 4, no. 2 (2009): 291–96.

———. "Stimulating Effect of Aromatherapy Massage with Jasmine Oil." *Natural Product Communications* 5, no. 1 (2010): 157–62.

Hongratanaworakit, T., and G. Buchbauer. "Relaxing Effect of Ylang Ylang Oil on Humans After Transdermal Absorption." *Phytotherapy Research* 20, no. 9 (2006): 758–63.

Huang, M. Y., M. H. Liao, Y. K. Wang, Y. S. Huang, and H. C. Wen. "Effect of Lavender Essential Oil on LPS-Stimulated Inflammation." *American Journal of Chinese Medicine* 40, no. 4 (2012): 845–59.

Hwang, J. H. "The Effects of the Inhalation Method Using Essential Oils on Blood Pressure and the Stress Response of Clients with Essential Hypertension." [In Korean.] *Taehan Kanho Hakhoe Chi* 36, no. 7 (2006): 1123–34.

Igarashi, M., H. Ikei, C. Song, and Y. Miyazaki. "Effects of Olfactory Stimulation with Rose and Orange Oil on Prefrontal Cortex Activity." *Complementary Therapies in Medicine* 22, no. 6 (2014): 1027–31.

Imanishi, J., H. Kuriyama, I. Shigemori, S. Watanabe, Y. Aihara, K. Masakazu, K. Sawai, H. Nakajima, N. Yoshida, M. Kunisawa, M. Kawase, and K. Fukui. "Anxiolytic Effect of Aromatherapy Massage in Patients with Breast Cancer." *Evidence-Based Complementary and Alternative Medicine* 6, no. 1 (2009): 123–28.

Jafarzadeh, M., S. Arman, and F. F. Pour. "Effect of Aromatherapy with Orange Essential Oil on Salivary Cortisol and Pulse Rate in Children During Dental Treatment: A Randomized Controlled Clinical Trial." *Advanced Biomedical Research* 2 (2013): 10.

Joanna Vargas Skin Care (blog). Accessed September 14, 2015. http://joannavargas.com /blog/.

Johnson, Scott A. *Surviving When Modern Medicine Fails: A Definitive Guide to Essential Oils That Could Save Your Life During a Crisis.* 2nd ed. n.p.: Scott A. Johnson, 2014.

Joseph, C. N., C. Porta, G. Casucci, N. Casiraghi, M. Maffeis, M. Rossi, and L. Bernardi. "Slow Breathing Improves Arteria Baroreflex Sensitivity and Decreases Blood Pressure in Essential Hypertension." *Hypertension* 46, no. 4 (2005): 714–18.

Juergens, U. R., U. Dethlefsen, G. Steinkamp, A. Gillissen, R. Repges, and H. Vetter. "Anti-inflammatory Activity of 1.8-Cineol (Eucalyptol) in Bronchial Asthma: A Double-Blind Placebo-Controlled Trial." *Respiratory Medicine* 97, no. 3 (2003): 250–56.

Kallor, A. "What You Need to Know Before You Get Your Nails Done." *Vogue.* May 13, 2015. http://www.vogue.com/13266401/jenna-hipp-nail-salon-safety/.

Karadag, E., S. Samancioglu, D. Ozden, and E. Bakir. "Effects of Aromatherapy on Sleep Quality and Anxiety of Patients." *Nursing in Critical Care.* July 27, 2015.

Kim, I.-H., C. Kim, K. Seong, M.-H. Hur, H. M. Lim, and M. S. Lee. "Essential Oil Inhalation on Blood Pressure and Salivary Cortisol Levels in Prehypertensive and Hypertensive Subjects." *Evidence-Based Complementary and Alternative Medicine* 2012 (2012): article ID 984203.

Kim, M. J., E. S. Nam, and S. I. Paik. "The Effects of Aromatherapy on Pain, Depression, and Life Satisfaction of Arthritis Patients." [In Korean.] *Taehan Kanho Hakhoe Chi* 35, no. 1 (2005): 186–94.

Koutroumanidou, E., A. Kimbaris, A. Kortsaris, E. Bezirtzoglou, M. Polissiou, K. Charalabopoulous, and O. Pagonopoulou. "Increased Seizure Latency and Decreased Severity in Pentylenetetrazol-Induced Seizures in Mice After Essential Oil Administration." *Epilepsy Research and Treatment* 2013 (2013): article ID 532657.

Kurtz, E. S., and W. Wallo. "Colloidal Oatmeal: History, Chemistry, and Clinical Properties." *Journal of Drugs in Dermatology* 6, no. 2 (2007): 167–70.

Lawless, Julia. *The Encyclopedia of Essential Oils: A Complete Guide to the Use of Aromatics in Aromatherapy, Herbalism, Health, and Well-Being.* Newburyport, MA: Conari Press, 1995.

Lazar, S. W., C. E. Kerr, R. H. Wasserman, J. R. Gray, D. N. Greve, M. T. Treadway, M. McGarvey, B. T. Quinn, J. A. Dusek, H. Benson, S. L. Rauch, C. I. Moore, and B. Fischl. "Meditation Experience Is Associated with Increased Cortical Thickness." *Neuroreport* 16, no. 17 (2005): 1893–97.

Lee, K. B., E. Cho, and K. S. Kang. "Changes in 5-Hydroxtryptamine and Cortisol Plasma Levels in Menopausal Women After Inhalation of Clary Sage Oil." *Phytotherapy Research* 28, no. 11 (2014): 1599–605.

Lis-Balchin, M. "Essential Oils and 'Aromatherapy': Their Modern Role in Healing." *Journal of the Royal Society of Health* 117, no. 5 (1997): 324–29.

Lv, X. N., Z. J. Liu, H. J. Zhang, and C. M. Tzeng. "Aromatherapy and the Central Nerve System (CNS): Therapeutic Mechanism and Its Associated Genes." *Current Drug Targets* 14, no. 8 (2013): 872–79.

Maldonado, M. C., M. P. Aban, and A. R. Navarro. "Chemicals and Lemon Essential Oil Effect on *Alicyclobacillus Acidoterrestris* Viability." *Brazilian Journal of Microbiology* 44, no. 4 (2013): 1133–37.

Marzouk, T., R. Barakat, A. Ragab, F. Badria, and A. Badawy. "Lavender-Thymol as a New Topical Aromatherapy Preparation for Episiotomy: A Randomised Clinical Trial." *Journal of Obstetrics and Gynaecology* 35, no. 5 (2015): 472–75.

Mojay, Gabriel. *Aromatherapy for Healing the Spirit: Restoring Emotional and Mental Balance with Essential Oils*. Rochester, VT: Healing Arts Press, 1999.

Mooney, C. "New Research Suggests Nature Walks Are Good for Your Brain." *Washington Post*. June 29, 2015. http://www.washingtonpost.com/news/energy-environment /wp/2015/06/29/fixating-or-brooding-on-things-take-a-walk-in-the-woods-for-real/.

Morris, Edwin T. *Scents of Time, Perfume from Ancient Egypt to 21st Century*. New York: Metropolitan Museum of Art; Boston: Bulfinch Press, 1999.

Naiafi, Z., M. Taghadosi, K. Sharifi, A. Farrokhian, and Z. Tagharrobi. "The Effects of Inhalation Aromatherapy on Anxiety in Patients with Myocardial Infarction: A Randomized Clinical Trial." *Iranian Red Crescent Medical Journal* 16, no. 8 (2014): e15485.

Ou, M. C., Y. F. Lee, C. C. Li, and S. K. Wu. "The Effectiveness of Essential Oils for Patients with Neck Pain: A Randomized Controlled Study." *Journal of Alternative and Complementary Medicine* 20, no. 10 (2014): 771–79.

Perry, N., and E. Perry. "Aromatherapy in the Management of Psychiatric Disorders: Clinical and Neuropharmacological Perspectives." *CNS Drugs* 20, no. 4 (2006): 257–80.

Price, Shirley, and Len Price. *Aromatherapy for Health Professionals*. 2nd ed. London: Elsevier Churchill Livingstone, 2002.

Purves, D., G. J. Augustine, D. Fitzpatrick, L. C. Katz, A.-S. LaMantia, J. O. McNamara, and S. M. Williams, eds. *Neuroscience*. 2nd ed. Sunderland, MA: Sinauer Associates, 2001.

Sadlon, A. E., and D. W. Lamson. "Immune-Modifying and Antimicrobial Effects of Eucalyptus Oil and Simple Inhalation Devices." *Alternative Medicine Review* 15, no. 1 (2010): 33–47.

Schnaubelt, Kurt. *Advanced Aromatherapy: The Science of Essential Oil Therapy*. Rochester, VT: Healing Arts Press, 1998.

———. *The Healing Intelligence of Essential Oils: The Science of Advanced Aromatherapy*. Rochester, VT: Healing Arts Press, 2011.

Shiina, Y., N. Funabashi, K. Lee, T. Toyoda, T. Sekine, S. Honjo, R. Hasegawa, T. Kawata, Y. Wakatsuki, S. Hayashi, S. Murakami, K. Koike, M. Daimon, and I. Komuro. "Relaxation Effects of Lavender Aromatherapy Improve Coronary Flow Velocity Reserve in Healthy Men Evaluated by Transthoracic Doppler Echocardiography." *International Journal of Cardiology* 129, no. 2 (2008): 193–97.

Slaughter, R. J., R. W. Mason, D. M. Beasley, J. A. Vale, and L. J. Schep. "Isopropanol Poisoning." *Clinical Toxicology* 52, no. 5 (2014): 470–78.

Su, H.-J., C.-J. Chao, H.-Y. Chang, and P.-C. Wu. "The Effects of Evaporating Essential Oils on Indoor Air Quality." *Atmospheric Environment* 41, no. 6 (2007): 1230–36.

Takahashi, M., A. Yamanaka, C. Asanuma, H. Asano, T. Satou, and K. Koike. "Anxiolytic-Like Effect of Inhalation of Essential Oil from Lavandula Officinalis: Investigation of Changes in 5-HT Turnover and Involvement of Olfactory Stimulation." *Natural Product Communications* 9, no. 7 (2014): 1023–26.

Tangel, K. "Morning Yoga While You 'Snooze': A Ten Minute Journey to Waking Up." *YinOva Center* (blog). Accessed September 14, 2015. https://www.yinovacenter.com/blog/morning-yoga-while-you-snooze-a-ten-minute-journey-to-waking-up/.

Tisserand, Robert. *Aromatherapy to Heal and Tend the Body*. Wilmot, WI: Lotus Press, 1988.

———. "Therapeutic Foundations of Essential Oils." Tisserand Institute webinar. June 2015. http://tisserandinstitute.org/available-webinars/.

Tisserand, R., and R. Young, *Essential Oil Safety: A Guide for Health Care Professionals*. 2nd ed. London: Churchill Livingstone Elsevier, 2014.

Veriditas Botanicals, http://veriditasbotanicals.com.

Wikipedia. "Nicholas Culpeper." Accessed September 14, 2015. https://en.wikipedia.org /wiki/Nicholas_Culpeper.

Willmont, Dennis. *Aromatherapy with Chinese Medicine: Healing the Body, Mind, Spirit with Essential Oils.* 3rd ed. Marshfield, MA: Willmountain Press, 2008.

Worwood, Valerie Ann. *The Complete Book of Essential Oils and Aromatherapy.* Novato, CA: New World Library, 1991.

Yuen, Jeffrey. *Materia Medica of Essential Oils: Based on a Chinese Medical Perspective.* New York: Ambrosia Press, 2008.

Zabirunnisa, M., J. S. Gadagi, P. Gadde, N. Myla, J. Koneru, and C. Thatimatla. "Dental Patient Anxiety: Possible Deal with Lavender Fragrance." *Journal of Research in Pharmacy Practice* 3, no. 3 (2014): 100–3.

Zabka, M., R. Pavela, and E. Prokinova. "Antifungal Activity and Chemical Composition of Twenty Essential Oils Against Significant Indoor and Outdoor Toxigenic and Aeroallergenic Fungi." *Chemosphere* 112 (October 2014): 443–48.

INDEX

*Page numbers in **bold** indicate the main description of the essential oil, blend, or term.*